EXPLORING PLASMODIUM OVALE

A COMPREHENSIVE GUIDE TO MALARIA'S LESSER-KNOWN CULPRIT

TOM WILES

DISCLAIMER

The information presented in this book is intended for general informational purposes only. The author and publisher have made every effort to ensure the accuracy of the information within this publication, but make no warranties or representations as to the accuracy, completeness, or suitability of the content. The information provided is subject to change without notice.

The author and publisher disclaim any liability, loss, or risk incurred as a consequence, directly or indirectly, of the use and application of any of the contents of this book. Readers are encouraged to consult with healthcare professionals, experts, and relevant authorities for specific medical or scientific advice and information.

The views and opinions expressed in this book are those of the author and do not necessarily reflect the official policy or position of any institution, organization, or entity mentioned herein.

TABLE OF CONTENT

INTRODUCTION

Welcome to the enthralling world of "Exploring Plasmodium Ovale – A Comprehensive Guide to Malaria's Lesser-Known Culprit" by Tom Wiles. It is with great pleasure that we invite you on a journey deep into the realms of one of nature's most elusive yet significant adversaries.

Malaria, a disease that has plagued humanity for centuries, is often associated with the notorious Plasmodium falciparum. However, there exists a lesser-known but equally intriguing culprit in the Malaria saga- Plasmodium ovale. With this book, Tom Wiles opens a door to the lesser-explored facets of this elusive parasite, unveiling its secrets, its impact, and the remarkable efforts being made to combat it.

As you delve into the pages of this comprehensive guide, you'll embark on a captivating voyage through the intricate biology of Plasmodium ovale, its life cycle, and its unique characteristics that distinguish it from its counterparts.

But this book is more than just a scientific exploration; it's a testament to the relentless pursuit of knowledge and the dedication of countless researchers, healthcare professionals, and advocates who strive to eradicate malaria from our world.

Tom Wiles, a seasoned expert in the field, masterfully combines scientific rigor with a passion for storytelling. He not only offers a deep understanding of Plasmodium ovale but also shares the stories of those on the frontlines of the battle against malaria, providing a human touch to the scientific narrative.

Whether you are a student seeking to expand your knowledge, a healthcare practitioner aiming to enhance your understanding, or simply a curious mind eager to learn, this book is a valuable resource. It bridges the gap between scientific complexity and accessibility, making the intricate world of malaria and Plasmodium ovale approachable to all.

We hope you find "Exploring Plasmodium Ovale" enlightening, inspiring, and thought-provoking

CHAPTER 1: INTRODUCTION TO PLASMODIUM OVALE

UNDERSTANDING THE DIVERSITY OF MALARIA PARASITES

Malaria, a global health challenge for centuries, is caused by a diverse group of parasitic organisms belonging to the genus Plasmodium. While most people are familiar with Plasmodium falciparum, the deadliest of these parasites, it is essential to recognize that malaria is not a one-size-fits-all disease. To truly grasp the complexity of malaria and develop effective strategies for its control and eradication, it is imperative to understand the diversity of malaria parasites.

At the heart of this diversity lie several distinct Plasmodium species, each with its own unique characteristics, life cycles, geographic distributions, and clinical manifestations. While the majority of human malaria cases are caused by P. falciparum and Plasmodium vivax, there are several other lesser-known species that contribute to the intricate tapestry of this disease, including Plasmodium malariae, Plasmodium ovale, and Plasmodium knowlesi.

Plasmodium falciparum: This species is notorious for its severe and often fatal manifestations. It is responsible for the majority of malaria-related deaths worldwide, particularly in sub-Saharan Africa. P. falciparum has a unique ability to adhere to and clog blood vessels, leading to severe complications such as cerebral malaria.

Plasmodium vivax: Although not as deadly as P. falciparum, P. vivax poses its own set of challenges. It has a dormant stage in the liver, causing relapses months or even years after the initial infection. This feature makes it particularly difficult to eliminate and contributes to the overall burden of malaria.

Plasmodium malariae: P. malariae is less common but is known for causing chronic, low-level infections that can persist for many years. It often goes undetected due to its less severe symptoms, but it can lead to long-term health issues.

Plasmodium ovale: Plasmodium ovale is a lesser-known member of the Plasmodium family. It is primarily found in Africa and is known for its oval-shaped red blood cell forms.

While typically less severe than P. falciparum, it can cause relapses similar to P. vivax, making it a challenging target for elimination.

Plasmodium knowlesi: Found in Southeast Asia, P. knowlesi is a malaria parasite that primarily infects macaque monkeys. However, it can also infect humans, leading to severe and sometimes fatal malaria. Its zoonotic nature presents unique challenges for malaria control in certain regions.

Understanding this diversity is not merely an academic pursuit but has profound implications for public health. Different Plasmodium species may require distinct diagnostic methods, treatment approaches, and control strategies. For instance, drugs effective against P. falciparum may not work against P. vivax due to differences in their biology. Moreover, vaccines targeting one species may not confer immunity against others.

Furthermore, the geographic distribution of these species varies, with some being more prevalent in certain regions.

This knowledge is crucial for tailoring interventions to specific areas and populations, ensuring the most effective use of limited resources.

The diversity of malaria parasites is a central facet of the malaria challenge. Recognizing and studying these differences is essential for advancing our understanding of the disease and for developing comprehensive and targeted approaches to malaria control and elimination. As we continue to confront this global health threat, we must embrace the complexity of malaria parasites and work collaboratively to combat each of them effectively, ultimately bringing us closer to a world free of malaria's burden.

HISTORICAL PERSPECTIVE ON MALARIA RESEARCH

The history of malaria research is a tapestry woven with scientific breakthroughs, medical innovations, and a relentless pursuit of understanding a disease that has plagued humanity for millennia. Examining the historical perspective on malaria research not only sheds light on the evolution of our knowledge but also highlights the dedication and determination of scientists and healthcare professionals in the battle against this ancient and formidable adversary.

Ancient Observations and Remedies:

Malaria's presence can be traced back thousands of years. Ancient civilizations, from the Greeks to the Romans, made observations about the disease's recurrent fevers and chills. The term "malaria" itself is derived from the Italian words "mala" (bad) and "aria" (air), reflecting the once-common belief that the disease was caused by foul air from marshes.

Early attempts at treatment ranged from herbal remedies to bloodletting, reflecting a lack of understanding of the disease's true cause.

It wasn't until the late 19th century that the connection between mosquitoes and malaria transmission was made by Sir Ronald Ross, an English physician. His discovery marked a turning point in malaria research and earned him the Nobel Prize in Physiology or Medicine in 1902.

The Search for Effective Treatments:

The understanding of malaria's parasitic nature deepened with the discovery of the malaria parasite in red blood cells by Charles Louis Alphonse Laveran in 1880. Shortly after, the life cycle of the parasite was elucidated by Giovanni Battista Grassi and others, further advancing our understanding of the disease.

The early 20th century saw the development of quinine and other antimalarial drugs, which became crucial in treating and managing malaria. Quinine, derived from the bark of the cinchona tree, was known for its efficacy against the Plasmodium parasite. However, its side effects and the emergence of drug resistance underscored the need for continued research into better treatments.

The DDT Era and Global Efforts:

During World War II, the insecticide DDT was deployed to combat malaria by controlling mosquito populations. This marked one of the earliest large-scale, global efforts to control the disease. While DDT was effective in reducing malaria transmission, concerns about environmental impacts and the development of insecticide resistance led to its eventual decline.

Advances in Molecular Biology:

In the latter half of the 20th century, the advent of molecular biology revolutionized malaria research. Scientists gained insights into the genetics of both the parasite and the mosquito vector. This knowledge paved the way for the development of new antimalarial drugs and the exploration of potential vaccines.

The Quest for a Malaria Vaccine:

One of the most significant challenges in malaria research has been the development of an effective vaccine. Researchers have made substantial progress, with vaccines like RTS, S/AS01 (Mosquirix) gaining approval for use in some regions.

While these vaccines offer hope, challenges remain in achieving long-lasting and widespread immunity.

The Fight Continues:

In the 21st century, the fight against malaria continues with renewed vigor. International organizations, governments, and research institutions collaborate on various fronts, from improving diagnostic tools to implementing bed net distribution programs. Efforts to combat drug resistance and develop new, more effective treatments persist.

As we reflect on the historical perspective of malaria research, it is clear that the journey has been marked by both triumphs and challenges. The resilience of scientists, healthcare workers, and communities affected by malaria has driven progress, but the complex nature of the disease demands ongoing dedication and innovation. With each new discovery, we move closer to the ultimate goal: a world free of the burden of malaria.

Significance of Plasmodium Ovale in Malaria Epidemiology

Malaria, a disease caused by various species of the Plasmodium parasite, has long been a significant global health concern. Among these parasites, Plasmodium falciparum and Plasmodium vivax have historically garnered the most attention due to their prevalence and the severity of their clinical manifestations. However, Plasmodium ovale, a lesser-known member of the Plasmodium family, plays a vital but often underappreciated role in malaria epidemiology. Understanding its significance is essential for a comprehensive approach to malaria control and elimination.

1. Geographic Distribution:

Plasmodium ovale exhibits a unique geographic distribution, primarily affecting regions of Africa and the Western Pacific. While it may not be as widespread as P. falciparum or P. vivax, its presence is notable.

This distribution has implications for local healthcare systems, as understanding which malaria species are prevalent in a given region is critical for accurate diagnosis and treatment.

2. Clinical Characteristics:

Plasmodium ovale infections typically present with milder clinical symptoms compared to P. falciparum. While this may suggest a lower public health threat, it is essential to recognize that even milder forms of malaria can have serious consequences, especially in vulnerable populations such as young children and pregnant women. Additionally, P. ovale is known for its ability to cause relapses, similar to P. vivax. These relapses can occur months or even years after the initial infection, adding complexity to case management and control efforts.

3. Diagnostic Challenges:

Accurate diagnosis is a cornerstone of effective malaria control. However, distinguishing P. ovale from other Plasmodium species can be challenging.

Traditional microscopy may not always differentiate between species accurately, and molecular diagnostic methods are often required. These challenges highlight the need for improved diagnostic tools and training for healthcare providers to ensure proper identification and treatment.

4. Genetic Diversity:

Plasmodium ovale exhibits genetic diversity, with distinct strains known as P. ovale curtisi and P. ovale wallikeri. Understanding this genetic diversity is crucial for tracking transmission patterns, detecting drug resistance, and developing targeted interventions.

5. Malaria Elimination Efforts:

In regions aiming to eliminate malaria, such as parts of Southeast Asia and the Western Pacific, P. ovale's ability to cause relapses poses challenges. Achieving elimination requires not only treating acute infections but also targeting dormant liver-stage parasites responsible for relapses. This demands a comprehensive approach that includes radical cure treatments.

6. Research and Vaccine Development:

Research on P. ovale is essential for advancing our understanding of its biology, transmission dynamics, and potential vulnerabilities. Additionally, as efforts to develop a malaria vaccine continue, it is crucial to consider P. ovale in vaccine design and evaluation, given its presence in malaria-endemic areas.

While Plasmodium ovale may not command the same attention as P. falciparum or P. vivax, its significance in malaria epidemiology should not be underestimated. Recognizing its distinct characteristics and geographic distribution is vital for accurate diagnosis, effective case management, and tailored control strategies. To achieve the ambitious goal of global malaria elimination, we must consider all species of malaria parasites, including P. ovale, and address the unique challenges they present.

CHAPTER 2: THE LIFE CYCLE UNVEILED

A DETAILED LOOK AT PLASMODIUM OVALE'S COMPLEX LIFE CYCLE

Plasmodium ovale, one of the lesser-known species responsible for causing malaria in humans, possesses a complex and fascinating life cycle that plays a critical role in its survival and transmission. To understand the intricacies of this parasite and develop effective strategies for its control, it is essential to take a closer look at the various stages of its life cycle.

1. Introduction to Plasmodium Ovale:

Plasmodium ovale is a protozoan parasite belonging to the Plasmodium genus, which includes several species responsible for causing malaria in humans. P. ovale is primarily found in certain regions of Africa and the Western Pacific and is responsible for a proportion of malaria cases in these areas.

2. The Life Cycle Begins:

The life cycle of Plasmodium ovale begins when an infected female Anopheles mosquito bites a human host.

During the blood meal, the mosquito injects sporozoites, a stage of the parasite, into the human's bloodstream.

3. Liver Stage Infection:

Once inside the human host, sporozoites travel to the liver, where they infect hepatocytes (liver cells). Unlike some other malaria parasites, P. ovale can remain dormant in the liver for extended periods, potentially causing relapses of the disease months or even years after the initial infection.

4. Release of Merozoites:

At a certain point, dormant forms of P. ovale, known as hypnozoites, can become active and develop into merozoites within hepatocytes. Merozoites are the next stage of the parasite's life cycle and are released into the bloodstream.

5. Blood Stage Infection:

Merozoites invade red blood cells, initiating the blood stage of the infection. Inside the red blood cells, P. ovale undergoes a series of transformations, replicating and multiplying.

This replication cycle is responsible for the characteristic symptoms of malaria, including fever, chills, and anemia.

6. Transmission to Mosquitoes:

When an infected mosquito bites a human host, it ingests the gametocytes, another stage of the parasite, from the host's bloodstream. Gametocytes are the sexual forms of the parasite.

7. Fertilization and Sporozoite Formation:

Inside the mosquito's gut, male and female gametocytes fuse, forming zygotes. These zygotes eventually develop into sporozoites, the same stage that initially infected the human host.

8. Migration to Salivary Glands:

The sporozoites then migrate to the mosquito's salivary glands, ready to be transmitted to another human host during a subsequent blood meal.

This complex life cycle of Plasmodium ovale, with its ability to persist in the liver as dormant forms, contributes to the challenges of diagnosing and treating the disease. It also underscores the importance of comprehensive treatment that targets both the acute blood stage infection and the dormant liver-stage parasites to prevent relapses.

Understanding the intricacies of the parasite's life cycle is crucial for the development of effective interventions, including drugs that can target the dormant liver forms and vaccines that can disrupt the transmission cycle. As research into malaria continues, a deeper understanding of Plasmodium ovale's life cycle promises to be a valuable tool in the ongoing efforts to control and ultimately eliminate this lesser-known but significant contributor to the global burden of malaria.

MOSQUITO HOSTS AND HUMAN HOSTS: A SYMBIOTIC RELATIONSHIP

In the intricate world of malaria, an ancient and devastating disease, a complex and symbiotic relationship exists between mosquito hosts and human hosts. This relationship, while seemingly adversarial, is fundamental to the perpetuation and transmission of the Plasmodium parasite, the causative agent of malaria. Understanding this intricate dance between mosquitoes and humans is pivotal in our efforts to combat this global health challenge.

Mosquitoes as Vectors:

Female Anopheles mosquitoes serve as vectors for the transmission of malaria. These mosquitoes are not inherently malicious; rather, they become unwitting carriers of the Plasmodium parasite when they feed on the blood of an infected human host. The parasite undergoes a crucial part of its life cycle within the mosquito.

Feeding on Human Blood:

The female Anopheles mosquito's quest for a blood meal to nourish her eggs brings her into contact with human hosts. During this feeding process, the mosquito injects saliva to prevent blood clotting. Simultaneously, it introduces Plasmodium sporozoites into the bloodstream of the human host. These sporozoites are the infectious stage of the parasite that travels to the liver and initiates the infection.

A Journey Through the Human Body:

Once inside the human host, Plasmodium undergoes several stages, ultimately infecting red blood cells and causing the symptoms associated with malaria. This is where the disease manifests, leading to fever, chills, fatigue, and, in severe cases, life-threatening complications.

Transmission Back to Mosquitoes:

The cycle continues when another female Anopheles mosquito feeds on an infected human host, ingesting gametocytes—the sexual stage of the parasite—from the bloodstream.

Inside the mosquito's gut, male and female gametocytes fuse, forming zygotes. These zygotes develop into sporozoites, which migrate to the mosquito's salivary glands, ready to infect another human host during the mosquito's next blood meal.

A Symbiotic Dance:

This intricate transmission cycle underscores the symbiotic relationship between mosquitoes and humans. While the Plasmodium parasite causes immense suffering in human hosts, mosquitoes serve as unwitting vehicles that allow the parasite to complete its life cycle. From an evolutionary perspective, this relationship has persisted because it benefits the parasite's survival and spread.

Implications for Malaria Control:

Understanding the symbiotic relationship between mosquitoes and humans is crucial for effective malaria control and prevention. Efforts to combat malaria often focus on interrupting this transmission cycle, whether through insecticide-treated bed nets, indoor residual spraying, or the development of vaccines.

By reducing the mosquito's ability to transmit the parasite, we can break the chain of transmission and reduce the burden of malaria.

Additionally, research into mosquito biology and genetics can yield insights into vector control strategies, such as the development of genetically modified mosquitoes that are less efficient at transmitting the parasite.

The interaction between mosquito hosts and human hosts in the context of malaria is a remarkable example of the complex relationships that exist in the natural world. While the disease itself is a significant global health challenge, understanding this symbiotic relationship is essential for our ongoing efforts to combat malaria and, ultimately, eliminate it as a public health threat.

DIFFERENTIATING PLASMODIUM OVALE FROM OTHER MALARIA PARASITES

While Plasmodium falciparum and Plasmodium vivax are the most well-known species, Plasmodium ovale, a less common but significant contributor to malaria cases, often goes unnoticed due to its relatively milder symptoms. Differentiating Plasmodium ovale from other malaria parasites is crucial for accurate diagnosis, appropriate treatment, and effective malaria control efforts.

Clinical Presentation:

One of the primary challenges in differentiating Plasmodium ovale from other malaria parasites lies in the clinical presentation. P. ovale infections tend to be less severe compared to P. falciparum, which can cause life-threatening complications. Symptoms of P. ovale infection often include fever, chills, headache, and muscle aches, which can overlap with the symptoms of other malaria species. However, P. ovale is distinctive in that it can cause relapses, similar to P. vivax.

Microscopic Examination:

Microscopic examination of blood smears remains a standard method for differentiating malaria species. Under a microscope, the appearance of the parasite's stages within red blood cells can offer clues. Plasmodium ovale typically exhibits an oval or elliptical shape, distinguishing it from the more circular forms of P. falciparum and P. vivax. Additionally, the presence of Schüffner's dots (small, dark dots within the red blood cells) is a characteristic feature of P. ovale.

Molecular Diagnostic Tools:

Advancements in molecular diagnostic techniques have significantly improved the accuracy of malaria species differentiation. Polymerase chain reaction (PCR) assays and rapid diagnostic tests (RDTs) targeting specific genetic markers can identify the Plasmodium species with a high degree of precision. Molecular tools are especially valuable in regions where multiple malaria species coexist, ensuring the correct identification of the infecting species.

Geographic Distribution:

Understanding the geographic distribution of malaria species can also aid in differentiation. P. ovale is primarily found in specific regions of Africa and the Western Pacific, whereas P. falciparum is prevalent in sub-Saharan Africa, and P. vivax is more widely distributed, including in South and Southeast Asia. Knowledge of the local epidemiology can provide initial insights into the likely malaria species.

Relapse Patterns:

Plasmodium ovale's unique feature of causing relapses can be diagnostically significant. If a patient with a previous P. ovale infection experiences recurrent malaria symptoms months or years after the initial episode, it may suggest a relapse rather than a new infection with a different species. This information can guide healthcare providers in tailoring treatment strategies.

Differentiating Plasmodium ovale from other malaria parasites is a critical aspect of malaria diagnosis and management.

Accurate identification ensures that patients receive appropriate treatment, preventing relapses and complications. Advances in diagnostic techniques, coupled with a comprehensive understanding of the clinical and epidemiological characteristics of each species, empower healthcare professionals to effectively combat malaria, regardless of the infecting parasite.

CHAPTER 3: GEOGRAPHIC DISTRIBUTION

GLOBAL DISTRIBUTION PATTERNS OF PLASMODIUM OVALE

Plasmodium ovale, one of the less common human malaria parasites, exhibits a distinct global distribution pattern that contributes to its unique epidemiology and significance in malaria research and control efforts. Understanding where Plasmodium ovale is prevalent is crucial for targeted interventions, accurate diagnosis, and effective malaria control.

1. Regions in Africa:

Plasmodium ovale is most frequently encountered in regions of sub-Saharan Africa, particularly in West Africa. Countries such as Nigeria, Ghana, Cameroon, and Liberia have reported a relatively high prevalence of P. ovale infections. Within these areas, the distribution of P. ovale can be further localized, varying from one region to another.

2. Western Pacific Islands:

In addition to its presence in Africa, P. ovale is also found in parts of the Western Pacific, including Indonesia and Papua New Guinea.

These areas have reported cases of P. ovale infections, though the prevalence may not be as high as in some African countries.

3. Variability Within Regions:

Even within regions where P. ovale is prevalent, there can be significant variability in its distribution. Factors such as climate, mosquito vector species, and human population movement can influence the local prevalence of this parasite. In some cases, it may be more common in rural areas, while in others, it may be found in both urban and rural settings.

4. Imported Cases:

In areas where P. ovale is not endemic, such as many parts of Europe and North America, cases of P. ovale infection often occur in travelers who have visited malaria-endemic regions. This highlights the importance of considering imported cases in non-endemic countries, as they can serve as a source of local transmission if appropriate mosquito vectors are present.

5. Co-Endemicity:

In regions where P. ovale is prevalent, it often coexists with other malaria parasite species, such as Plasmodium falciparum and Plasmodium vivax. Co-endemicity of multiple Plasmodium species presents diagnostic and treatment challenges, as each species may require specific approaches for accurate diagnosis and effective management.

6. Changing Distribution Patterns:

The distribution of Plasmodium ovale, like other malaria parasites, can change over time due to various factors, including climate change, population movement, and control interventions. Surveillance efforts are essential for monitoring these changes and adapting malaria control strategies accordingly.

Understanding the global distribution patterns of Plasmodium ovale is vital for healthcare systems and researchers. It informs the choice of diagnostic methods, treatment regimens, and vector control strategies.

As we continue to combat malaria and work toward its eventual elimination, a comprehensive understanding of the geographic distribution of all malaria species, including P. ovale, remains essential to achieving the goal of a malaria-free world.

FACTORS INFLUENCING GEOGRAPHIC PREVALENCE

The geographic prevalence of malaria parasites, including Plasmodium species such as Plasmodium ovale, is influenced by a complex interplay of various factors. Understanding these factors is crucial for predicting and managing the distribution of malaria parasites and for implementing effective control measures. Here, we explore some of the key factors that influence the geographic prevalence of malaria parasites.

1. Climate and Temperature:

Malaria transmission is highly sensitive to temperature and climatic conditions. Anopheles mosquitoes, the primary vectors of malaria, thrive in warm and humid environments. Temperature affects both the development of the malaria parasite within the mosquito and the lifespan and behavior of the mosquito vector. Hence, regions with consistently warm temperatures are more conducive to malaria transmission, leading to higher prevalence.

2. Rainfall and Water Bodies:

Rainfall patterns also play a crucial role in malaria prevalence. Prolonged rainy seasons create stagnant water bodies, which serve as breeding grounds for mosquito larvae. An increase in suitable breeding sites can lead to an upsurge in mosquito populations and subsequent malaria transmission. Conversely, areas with limited rainfall may have fewer breeding sites and lower malaria prevalence.

3. Altitude and Topography:

Altitude and topography significantly influence malaria prevalence. In many cases, malaria transmission decreases with increasing altitude. This is due to lower temperatures and reduced mosquito populations at higher elevations. Mountainous regions often have lower malaria burdens compared to lowland areas.

4. Human Population Density:

The density and distribution of human populations are critical determinants of malaria prevalence.

Areas with dense populations, especially in urban and peri-urban settings, often experience higher transmission rates due to the higher likelihood of human-mosquito contact. Human migration patterns also impact the spread of malaria.

5. Vector Species and Behavior:

The presence of competent mosquito vector species is a key factor in malaria transmission. Different mosquito species exhibit varying degrees of competence in transmitting Plasmodium parasites. Additionally, mosquito behavior, such as feeding habits and resting preferences, can influence the efficiency of transmission.

6. Socioeconomic Factors:

Socioeconomic conditions, including poverty, access to healthcare, and housing quality, can affect malaria prevalence. Impoverished communities with limited access to healthcare may face higher malaria burdens due to a lack of preventative measures and inadequate treatment options.

7. Malaria Control Interventions:

The implementation of malaria control interventions, such as insecticide-treated bed nets, indoor residual spraying, and access to antimalarial drugs, can significantly reduce transmission and prevalence. The effectiveness and coverage of these interventions vary by region and can impact malaria patterns.

8. Environmental Changes:

Human-induced environmental changes, such as deforestation, urbanization, and land use alterations, can alter the natural habitats of mosquitoes and influence the distribution of malaria parasites. Changes in land use can create new breeding sites or disrupt existing ones.

9. Climate Change:

Long-term climate changes can have profound effects on malaria prevalence. Altered rainfall patterns, temperature shifts, and changes in the geographic distribution of mosquito vectors can result from climate change, potentially expanding the range of malaria transmission.

10. Human Behavior and Travel:

Human behavior, including travel and migration, can introduce malaria parasites to new areas. Travelers returning from malaria-endemic regions can carry the parasite to non-endemic areas, leading to localized outbreaks.

The geographic prevalence of malaria parasites, such as Plasmodium ovale, is the result of a complex interplay among climate, environmental factors, human behavior, vector characteristics, and control efforts. Monitoring and understanding these factors are essential for targeted malaria control strategies and the eventual goal of reducing and eliminating malaria worldwide.

IMPLICATIONS FOR MALARIA CONTROL AND ELIMINATION EFFORTS

Malaria, a global health challenge, remains a significant burden in many parts of the world. Effective control and eventual elimination of malaria require a deep understanding of the disease's dynamics, including its transmission patterns, geographic distribution, and the species of malaria parasites involved. In the case of Plasmodium ovale, recognizing its implications is crucial for tailored malaria control and elimination efforts.

1. Targeted Diagnostics:

Accurate diagnosis is the first step in effective malaria control. Identifying the specific Plasmodium species causing infections, including P. ovale, enables healthcare providers to prescribe appropriate antimalarial treatment regimens. Improved diagnostic tools that can differentiate between malaria species, such as molecular assays and rapid diagnostic tests, are essential in regions where multiple species coexist.

2. Treatment Strategies:

Plasmodium ovale's unique feature of causing relapses necessitates tailored treatment strategies. Radical cure, which targets both the acute blood-stage infection and the dormant liver forms (hypnozoites), is crucial to prevent relapses. Antimalarial drugs with activity against hypnozoites, such as primaquine, must be used judiciously, taking into account factors like glucose-6-phosphate dehydrogenase (G6PD) deficiency prevalence.

3. Vector Control:

Malaria vector control efforts, such as the use of insecticide-treated bed nets and indoor residual spraying, should be guided by the knowledge of local vector species and their behaviors. In regions where P. ovale is prevalent, it is essential to address potential vector breeding sites and maintain high coverage of vector control measures to reduce transmission.

4. Surveillance and Monitoring:

Robust surveillance systems are crucial for tracking malaria cases and understanding local transmission dynamics. Identifying areas with a high prevalence of P. ovale and monitoring changes in transmission patterns is essential for targeted interventions. Data on relapse cases should also be systematically collected and analyzed.

5. Cross-Border Collaboration:

In regions with mobile populations, cross-border collaboration is essential for malaria control. Migrants and travelers can introduce the parasite to new areas. Regional coordination ensures that control measures, diagnostics, and treatment are consistent and effective in preventing the spread of malaria.

6. Research and Vaccine Development:

Investment in research, including studies specific to P. ovale, is crucial for advancing our understanding of this parasite's biology and transmission. Additionally, as efforts to develop a malaria vaccine continue, it is vital to consider P. ovale in vaccine design and evaluation.

7. Community Engagement and Education:

Engaging communities and educating individuals about malaria prevention, diagnosis, and treatment is vital. Culturally sensitive outreach and education programs can increase awareness and encourage behavior changes that reduce malaria risk.

8. Global Malaria Elimination Initiatives:

The global community has set ambitious goals for malaria elimination. Plasmodium ovale, while often overshadowed by other species, must not be overlooked in these efforts. Tailoring elimination strategies to account for the presence of P. ovale in specific regions is essential for achieving these goals.

Plasmodium ovale's role in malaria epidemiology has significant implications for malaria control and elimination efforts. Recognizing the unique features of this parasite and its distribution patterns is essential for precision in diagnostics, treatment, vector control, and surveillance. As the world continues to work toward the ultimate goal of malaria elimination, comprehensive strategies that consider the diversity of malaria parasites, including P. ovale, are key to success.

CHAPTER 4: CLINICAL MANIFESTATIONS

UNMASKING PLASMODIUM OVALE'S CLINICAL PROFILE

In the realm of malaria parasites, Plasmodium ovale often remains shrouded in relative obscurity compared to its more infamous counterparts like Plasmodium falciparum and Plasmodium vivax. Yet, Plasmodium ovale is far from a minor player in the world of malaria. Unmasking its clinical profile is crucial for a comprehensive understanding of the disease and effective patient management.

1. Clinical Presentation:

Plasmodium ovale infections typically manifest with clinical symptoms similar to other malaria species, such as fever, chills, headache, fatigue, and muscle aches. These symptoms can often be nonspecific and overlap with those of other infectious diseases, making accurate diagnosis challenging.

2. Relapse Potential:

One of the distinguishing features of Plasmodium ovale is its capacity to cause relapses. Similar to Plasmodium vivax, P. ovale has hypnozoites, dormant forms of the parasite that can remain in the liver for extended periods. These hypnozoites can reactivate months or even years after the initial infection, leading to recurrent malaria episodes. The propensity for relapses necessitates specific treatment strategies to target both the acute infection and the dormant forms.

3. Severity Profile:

Plasmodium ovale infections generally tend to be less severe compared to those caused by Plasmodium falciparum, which can lead to severe complications, including cerebral malaria. However, it is important to recognize that even P. ovale infections can lead to severe outcomes, especially in vulnerable populations such as young children, pregnant women, or individuals with compromised immune systems.

4. Diagnosis Challenges:

Accurate diagnosis of Plasmodium ovale infections is a critical but challenging aspect of patient management. Traditional microscopy may not always distinguish between malaria species accurately. Molecular diagnostic methods, such as polymerase chain reaction (PCR) assays, offer higher specificity and sensitivity in identifying P. ovale infections.

5. Geographic Distribution:

Plasmodium ovale's distribution is primarily concentrated in specific regions of Africa and the Western Pacific. Knowledge of its geographic distribution is valuable for healthcare providers, enabling them to consider P. ovale as a potential cause of malaria in patients from these areas.

6. Treatment Approaches:

Effective treatment of P. ovale infections involves not only addressing the acute blood-stage infection but also targeting the dormant liver forms (hypnozoites) to prevent relapses.

Antimalarial drugs with activity against hypnozoites, such as primaquine, are essential components of treatment regimens.

7. Immunity and Research:

The clinical profile of Plasmodium ovale and its relapse potential raise intriguing questions about the development of immunity to this parasite and the interactions between acute and relapse episodes. Research into these aspects is essential for a deeper understanding of P. ovale's biology and for the development of effective control strategies.

Unmasking Plasmodium ovale's clinical profile is crucial for recognizing its unique characteristics, including the potential for relapses. A more comprehensive understanding of this lesser-known malaria species is essential for healthcare providers, researchers, and public health experts to tailor diagnosis, treatment, and control measures effectively. As the global effort to combat malaria continues, acknowledging the significance of Plasmodium ovale is a vital step toward a malaria-free future.

SYMPTOMS, DIAGNOSIS, AND CHALLENGES IN DETECTION

Plasmodium ovale, one of the lesser-known human malaria parasites, presents unique challenges in its diagnosis due to its clinical characteristics and the limitations of available diagnostic tools. Understanding the symptoms, diagnostic methods, and the challenges in detecting P. ovale is crucial for accurate diagnosis and effective management.

Symptoms:

Plasmodium ovale infections share common symptoms with other malaria parasites and typically include:

Fever: Fever is often the first and most prominent symptom, with intermittent spikes corresponding to the cyclic nature of malaria parasites.

Chills: Patients may experience cold shivers and chills during the fever episodes.

Headache: Headaches are common and can range from mild to severe.

Muscle Aches: Patients often complain of muscle pain and weakness.

Fatigue: A general sense of weakness and fatigue can persist between fever episodes.

Sweating: Profuse sweating often follows fever spikes.

Enlarged Spleen: In some cases, an enlarged spleen (splenomegaly) may be palpable on physical examination.

It is important to note that while P. ovale infections can cause discomfort and illness, they are generally less severe than infections with Plasmodium falciparum, the most dangerous malaria species.

Diagnosis:

Accurate diagnosis of Plasmodium ovale malaria is essential for appropriate treatment. Several diagnostic methods are available:

Microscopy: Traditionally, microscopic examination of blood smears has been the gold standard for malaria diagnosis.

P. ovale appears as oval or elliptical-shaped parasites within red blood cells, often with Schüffner's dots. However, microscopy may not always differentiate P. ovale from other species accurately.

Rapid Diagnostic Tests (RDTs): RDTs are simple, quick, and widely used diagnostic tools that detect specific malaria antigens in a patient's blood. While RDTs are convenient and useful in many settings, they may not always differentiate between malaria species.

Molecular Diagnostics: Polymerase chain reaction (PCR) assays and nucleic acid amplification tests (NAATs) are highly sensitive and specific molecular methods that can identify and differentiate Plasmodium species, including P. ovale.

Challenges in Detection:

Several challenges complicate the detection of Plasmodium ovale:

Similar Symptoms: The clinical symptoms of P. ovale malaria overlap with those of other malaria species, making it challenging to diagnose based solely on clinical presentation.

Microscopy Limitations: Microscopy relies on the skill of the technician and may not always distinguish P. ovale from other species accurately. Furthermore, it may not detect low-level parasitemia.

Access to Molecular Diagnostics: PCR and NAATs, while highly accurate, require specialized equipment and trained personnel, limiting their availability in resource-constrained settings.

Relapses: Plasmodium ovale's unique feature of causing relapses further complicates diagnosis. Relapses can occur months or even years after the initial infection, requiring a high degree of suspicion and appropriate treatment.

Co-Infections: Co-infections with multiple Plasmodium species can occur, further challenging species-specific diagnosis.

Diagnosing Plasmodium ovale malaria requires a combination of clinical suspicion and appropriate diagnostic tools. While traditional microscopy and

RDTs remain valuable, molecular diagnostics like PCR offer the highest specificity.

Addressing the challenges in detection, especially in regions where P. ovale is prevalent, is essential for accurate diagnosis and effective management of this lesser-known malaria species.

COMPARING CLINICAL FEATURES WITH OTHER MALARIA SPECIES

Malaria is a complex disease caused by various species of the Plasmodium parasite. Each species exhibits distinct clinical characteristics, including the severity of symptoms and potential complications. Plasmodium ovale, while less common than some other species like Plasmodium falciparum and Plasmodium vivax, has unique clinical features that set it apart from its counterparts.

Clinical Features of Plasmodium Ovale:

Fever: Like other malaria species, Plasmodium ovale infections typically present with fever. Fever in P. ovale infections can be cyclic, with recurring episodes of high temperature.

Chills and Sweats: Patients with P. ovale malaria often experience chills and profuse sweating, especially during fever episodes.

Headache: Headaches are a common symptom and can vary in intensity.

Muscle Aches: Muscle pain and weakness are typical and can contribute to overall discomfort.

Fatigue: A general sense of weakness and fatigue is common, especially during and after fever episodes.

Enlarged Spleen: In some cases, an enlarged spleen (splenomegaly) may be palpable on physical examination.

Comparison with Other Malaria Species:

Now, let's compare these clinical features with those of other prominent malaria species:

Plasmodium falciparum: This species is known for causing the most severe form of malaria. Symptoms can include high fever, severe anemia, organ dysfunction, and complications such as cerebral malaria. P. falciparum infections require prompt medical attention due to their potential for rapid progression.

Plasmodium vivax: Similar to P. ovale, P. vivax infections can cause relapses due to the presence of hypnozoites.

Symptoms are generally less severe than P. falciparum but can include fever, chills, headache, and muscle pain. P. vivax can also lead to complications, especially when relapses occur.

Plasmodium malariae: Infections with P. malariae tend to have a chronic course with less severe symptoms. Fever episodes may be less frequent, and the overall clinical picture can be milder. P. malariae is associated with persistent low-level parasitemia and can lead to kidney-related complications in the long term.

Mixed Infections: In regions where multiple Plasmodium species coexist, patients can experience mixed infections, where two or more species of the parasite are present simultaneously. This can complicate clinical presentation and diagnosis.

It's important to note that the clinical features of malaria can vary depending on factors such as the patient's age, immunity, and any underlying health conditions. Additionally, accurate diagnosis and appropriate treatment are essential for managing malaria effectively, as the choice of treatment may differ based on the infecting species.

Plasmodium ovale, while less severe compared to P. falciparum, shares some clinical features with other malaria species. However, its unique ability to cause relapses sets it apart and requires specific treatment strategies to target the dormant liver forms. Recognizing these differences is crucial for accurate diagnosis and appropriate patient management.

CHAPTER 5: MOLECULAR INSIGHTS

GENOMIC DISCOVERIES AND GENETIC VARIABILITY

The genomic exploration of Plasmodium ovale, one of the lesser-known malaria parasites, has unveiled valuable insights into its biology, evolution, and genetic diversity. These discoveries have far-reaching implications for understanding its epidemiology, drug resistance, and potential vaccine development.

1. Genomic Sequencing:

Advancements in genomics have enabled the sequencing of Plasmodium ovale genomes. By unraveling its genetic code, researchers have gained a deeper understanding of the parasite's biology. Comparative genomics with other Plasmodium species has provided insights into the unique features of P. ovale.

2. Species Differentiation:

Genomic analysis has allowed for precise species differentiation within the Plasmodium genus.

This is crucial in regions with multiple malaria species coexisting, ensuring accurate diagnosis and appropriate treatment.

3. Genetic Diversity:

Plasmodium ovale exhibits genetic diversity, which can impact the parasite's virulence, drug resistance, and transmission dynamics. Studies have identified various genetic variants, providing valuable information about the parasite's adaptability.

4. Drug Resistance:

Genomic studies have revealed the genetic markers associated with drug resistance in P. ovale. Understanding these markers is essential for monitoring and addressing resistance to antimalarial drugs, such as chloroquine.

5. Relapse Mechanisms:

Genomic research has shed light on the mechanisms underlying relapses in P. ovale infections. This includes identifying the genes responsible for the formation and activation of hypnozoites, the dormant liver-stage parasites that lead to relapses.

6. Host-Parasite Interactions:

Genomics has allowed for the exploration of host-parasite interactions at the molecular level. Understanding how P. ovale interacts with the human host's immune system can inform vaccine development efforts.

7. Vaccine Candidates:

Genomic insights have aided in the identification of potential vaccine candidates. Researchers are exploring proteins and antigens unique to P. ovale that could be targeted by vaccines to prevent infection or relapses.

8. Molecular Epidemiology:

Genomic tools are valuable for molecular epidemiology studies, tracking the spread and genetic diversity of P. ovale strains. This information is critical for designing effective malaria control strategies.

9. Evolutionary History:

Comparative genomics with other Plasmodium species has provided insights into the evolutionary history of P. ovale. Understanding its phylogenetic relationships can illuminate its origins and historical transmission patterns.

10. Future Research Avenues:

Genomic discoveries in Plasmodium ovale continue to open up new research avenues. Ongoing studies may reveal further details about its biology, transmission dynamics, and potential vulnerabilities.

Genomic research has played a pivotal role in advancing our understanding of Plasmodium ovale, shedding light on its genetic diversity, drug resistance, and relapse mechanisms. These insights are crucial for malaria control and elimination efforts and offer hope for the development of targeted interventions, including vaccines, to combat this lesser-known malaria parasite.

DRUG RESISTANCE AND ITS IMPLICATIONS

Drug resistance is a significant concern in the fight against malaria, including infections caused by Plasmodium ovale. Understanding the development of drug resistance, its implications for treatment, and strategies to address it is crucial for effective malaria control efforts.

1. Emergence of Drug Resistance:

Plasmodium ovale, like other malaria parasites, has demonstrated the capacity to develop resistance to antimalarial drugs over time. Resistance typically arises due to genetic mutations within the parasite population.

2. Chloroquine Resistance:

Chloroquine, once an effective treatment for P. ovale infections, has seen increasing resistance in some regions. Genetic studies have identified specific mutations in the parasite's chloroquine resistance transporter (PfCRT) gene associated with reduced drug susceptibility.

3. Implications for Treatment:

Drug resistance in P. ovale poses significant challenges for treatment. Resistant strains may not respond adequately to standard antimalarial medications, leading to treatment failures and persistent infections. This can result in prolonged illness and an increased risk of complications.

4. Increased Relapse Risk:

In cases of P. ovale infection, where relapses occur due to dormant liver-stage parasites (hypnozoites), drug resistance can complicate matters. Resistant strains may persist in the liver, leading to recurrent relapses even after successful treatment of the acute blood-stage infection.

5. Diagnostic Challenges:

Drug-resistant P. ovale strains may not be distinguishable from susceptible strains based solely on clinical symptoms or standard diagnostic methods. Molecular tests are required to identify specific drug resistance markers, adding complexity to diagnosis.

6. Spread of Resistance:

The spread of drug-resistant P. ovale strains within and between regions is a concern. Travelers and migrants can introduce resistant strains to new areas, potentially leading to localized outbreaks and complicating malaria control efforts.

7. Alternative Treatment Options:

In response to drug resistance, healthcare providers must turn to alternative antimalarial drugs. Options include artemisinin-based combination therapies (ACTs) and other medications like primaquine for targeting hypnozoites. However, the choice of alternative drugs depends on local resistance patterns and individual patient factors.

8. Monitoring and Surveillance:

Efforts to combat drug resistance in P. ovale and other malaria parasites rely on robust monitoring and surveillance systems.

Regular assessments of treatment efficacy and the genetic profile of parasite populations are essential to detect and respond to resistance promptly.

9. Combination Therapies:

Combination therapies, such as ACTs, are often used to treat malaria. These combinations of drugs with different mechanisms of action reduce the risk of resistance development and improve treatment effectiveness.

10. Research and Development:

Research into new antimalarial drugs and strategies is ongoing. The goal is to develop novel treatments that are not only effective but also less prone to resistance.

Drug resistance in Plasmodium ovale poses significant challenges for malaria treatment and control. It underscores the importance of a multifaceted approach, including surveillance, the use of combination therapies, and ongoing research to stay ahead of emerging resistance.

Timely detection and management of drug-resistant strains are critical to ensure effective treatment and reduce the burden of P. ovale malaria.

THE ROLE OF MOLECULAR BIOLOGY IN MALARIA RESEARCH

Malaria, caused by various Plasmodium species, remains a global health challenge. Molecular biology plays a pivotal role in advancing our understanding of the parasite's biology, transmission, drug resistance, and the development of effective control strategies. Here, we explore the critical role of molecular biology in malaria research.

1. Species Identification:

Molecular techniques, such as polymerase chain reaction (PCR) assays, allow for the accurate identification and differentiation of Plasmodium species. This is crucial in regions where multiple species coexist, ensuring appropriate treatment and control measures.

2. Drug Resistance Monitoring:

Molecular biology is essential for monitoring drug resistance in malaria parasites.

Researchers can identify genetic markers associated with resistance, enabling surveillance and the development of effective treatment regimens.

3. Genome Sequencing:

The sequencing of Plasmodium genomes has provided valuable insights into the parasite's biology and evolution. Comparative genomics with other species has revealed genes responsible for drug resistance, virulence factors, and vaccine candidates.

4. Study of Vector-Parasite Interactions:

Molecular biology allows scientists to investigate the complex interactions between malaria parasites and their mosquito vectors. Understanding the molecular basis of transmission is critical for vector control strategies.

5. Hypnozoite Detection:

Detection of hypnozoites, the dormant liver-stage forms of Plasmodium, is possible through molecular methods. This is particularly important for species like Plasmodium vivax and Plasmodium ovale, which can cause relapses.

6. Immunology Research:

Molecular biology helps unravel the intricacies of host-parasite interactions at the molecular level. This knowledge informs vaccine development efforts by identifying key parasite antigens and immune responses.

7. Epidemiology Studies:

Molecular epidemiology allows researchers to track the spread and genetic diversity of malaria parasites. It provides insights into transmission dynamics, helping design targeted interventions.

8. Drug Development:

Molecular biology contributes to the discovery and development of new antimalarial drugs. Targeting specific molecular pathways in the parasite can lead to the development of more effective and less toxic medications.

9. Vaccine Development:

Molecular approaches are integral to vaccine development against malaria. Identifying antigens that elicit protective immune responses and designing subunit vaccines are key components of malaria vaccine research.

10. Diagnosis and Point-of-Care Tests:

Molecular techniques have led to the development of highly sensitive and specific diagnostic tests, including nucleic acid-based tests. These tests are valuable in detecting low-level parasitemia and tracking drug resistance markers.

11. Genetic Modification for Research:

Genetic manipulation of malaria parasites in the laboratory, enabled by molecular techniques, allows researchers to study specific genes and their functions. This aids in understanding parasite biology and potential drug targets.

Molecular biology is a cornerstone of malaria research, driving advancements in diagnostics, treatment, control strategies, and vaccine development.

It empowers scientists to unravel the complex biology of Plasmodium parasites, ultimately contributing to the global effort to combat malaria and work towards its elimination.

CHAPTER 6: EPIDEMIOLOGY AND TRANSMISSION DYNAMICS

TRANSMISSION PATHWAYS AND VECTOR BIOLOGY

Malaria, a vector-borne disease caused by Plasmodium parasites, is primarily transmitted to humans through the bites of infected female Anopheles mosquitoes. Understanding the intricacies of transmission pathways and the biology of these mosquito vectors is crucial for malaria control and prevention efforts.

Transmission Pathways:

Mosquito-Borne Transmission: The most common mode of malaria transmission is through the bite of an infected female Anopheles mosquito. When a mosquito feeds on an infected human, it ingests Plasmodium parasites along with the blood. These parasites develop and multiply within the mosquito's body, eventually migrating to the mosquito's salivary glands. When the mosquito subsequently bites another human, it injects sporozoites (infectious forms of the parasite) into the person's bloodstream, initiating a new infection.

Vertical Transmission: In some cases, Plasmodium parasites can be transmitted from an infected pregnant woman to her unborn child. This is known as congenital or vertical transmission. Although relatively rare compared to mosquito-borne transmission, it can occur when the mother has a high level of parasites in her bloodstream.

Blood Transfusions: Malaria can be transmitted through blood transfusions when donated blood contains viable Plasmodium parasites. Blood banks and healthcare facilities in malaria-endemic regions must screen blood donations to prevent transfusion-associated infections.

Organ Transplants: In rare cases, organ transplants involving organs or tissues from individuals with latent or low-level Plasmodium infections can lead to malaria transmission to the transplant recipient.

Vector Biology:

Understanding the biology of Anopheles mosquitoes, the primary vectors of malaria, is crucial for effective malaria control:

Species Diversity: Anopheles mosquitoes encompass a diverse group of species, each with varying preferences for breeding sites, feeding behaviors, and vectorial capacity (the ability to transmit the parasite). The distribution of different Anopheles species varies by region and contributes to malaria epidemiology.

Breeding Sites: Anopheles mosquitoes lay their eggs in various aquatic habitats, such as stagnant water bodies, rice fields, and even artificial containers. Effective mosquito control often involves targeting these breeding sites to reduce mosquito populations.

Feeding Habits: Female Anopheles mosquitoes require blood meals to nourish their eggs. Different species may exhibit different feeding behaviors, including nighttime biting (nocturnal) or daytime biting (diurnal). Targeting mosquito feeding patterns can inform control strategies.

Vector Control: Implementing vector control measures, such as insecticide-treated bed nets and indoor residual spraying, is essential for reducing mosquito-human contact and interrupting malaria transmission. The choice of control methods depends on the local vector species and their behaviors.

Insecticide Resistance: Some Anopheles mosquito populations have developed resistance to commonly used insecticides. Monitoring and managing insecticide resistance are critical to maintain the effectiveness of vector control interventions.

Human-Mosquito Interactions: Human behaviors, such as sleeping habits, outdoor activities, and use of protective measures, can influence the risk of mosquito bites and subsequent malaria transmission. Health education and community engagement play a role in promoting preventive behaviors.

Understanding the transmission pathways and vector biology of malaria is fundamental for malaria control and elimination efforts. Targeted interventions that consider local vector species, their behaviors, and the dynamics of human-mosquito interactions are essential in reducing the burden of this mosquito-borne disease.

SURVEILLANCE STRATEGIES AND EPIDEMIOLOGICAL STUDIES

Effective surveillance and epidemiological studies are essential components of malaria control programs. They provide critical insights into the distribution of the disease, its transmission dynamics, and the impact of control measures. Here, we explore the key surveillance strategies and epidemiological studies that underpin malaria control efforts.

1. Passive Surveillance:

Passive surveillance relies on healthcare facilities and local health systems to report cases of malaria as they occur. It is a foundational component of monitoring the disease burden and detecting outbreaks. Passive surveillance is useful for tracking individual cases and treatment outcomes.

2. Active Surveillance:

Active surveillance involves proactively seeking out and testing individuals for malaria, often through house-to-house visits, mobile clinics, or community health workers.

This approach is particularly valuable in regions with low transmission rates or in post-elimination phases.

3. Case Notification and Reporting:

Timely and accurate case notification and reporting are critical for surveillance. Healthcare providers, laboratories, and public health authorities must promptly report malaria cases to a central database, allowing for real-time monitoring and response.

4. Epidemiological Surveys:

Cross-sectional surveys, longitudinal cohort studies, and prevalence surveys are used to estimate the prevalence of malaria in specific populations. These surveys help identify high-risk groups and assess the impact of control measures.

5. Entomological Surveillance:

Entomological surveillance focuses on monitoring mosquito vectors and their behavior. This includes tracking vector abundance, species composition, insecticide resistance, and mosquito breeding sites. Understanding vector dynamics is vital for targeted vector control.

6. Malaria Indicator Surveys (MIS):

MIS are comprehensive household surveys that collect data on malaria prevalence, interventions (such as bed net use and indoor spraying), and access to malaria treatment. They provide valuable information for program evaluation and decision-making.

7. Sentinel Site Surveillance:

Sentinel site surveillance involves monitoring specific healthcare facilities or geographic locations that are representative of larger populations. This approach can provide early warning of outbreaks and trends.

8. Epidemiological Modeling:

Mathematical modeling techniques are used to simulate malaria transmission dynamics, predict future trends, and evaluate the potential impact of interventions. Models help guide decision-making and resource allocation.

9. Genomic Epidemiology:

Advancements in molecular biology allow for the genetic characterization of malaria parasites.

Genomic epidemiology helps trace the source of infections, detect drug resistance, and understand transmission patterns.

10. Geographic Information Systems (GIS):

GIS technology is used to map the spatial distribution of malaria cases, vector breeding sites, and control interventions. Spatial analysis informs the targeting of resources and interventions in specific geographic areas.

11. Surveillance for Imported Cases:

In regions where malaria is not endemic, surveillance for imported cases is crucial. Identifying and treating cases among travelers and migrants helps prevent local transmission and outbreaks.

12. Program Evaluation:

Epidemiological studies and surveillance data are used to assess the impact of malaria control programs and guide adjustments to strategies and interventions.

Surveillance strategies and epidemiological studies are fundamental tools in the fight against malaria.

They provide the data necessary for evidence-based decision-making, enabling targeted interventions, monitoring progress, and ultimately working toward the goal of malaria elimination.

TARGETED INTERVENTIONS FOR PLASMODIUM OVALE CONTROL

While Plasmodium ovale is often overshadowed by its more virulent malaria counterparts, it is essential to implement targeted interventions to control and eliminate this lesser-known parasite effectively. Tailoring strategies for P. ovale control involves understanding its unique features, such as relapse potential, geographic distribution, and treatment challenges. Here are key targeted interventions for P. ovale control:

1. Accurate Diagnosis:

Molecular Diagnostics: Utilize molecular diagnostic tools like polymerase chain reaction (PCR) assays to accurately identify and differentiate P. ovale from other malaria species. Molecular tests are particularly valuable in regions with mixed infections.

2. Effective Treatment Strategies:

Radical Cure: Plasmodium ovale's ability to cause relapses necessitates radical cure.

Administer antimalarial drugs with activity against hypnozoites, such as primaquine, in addition to drugs that treat the acute blood-stage infection. Consider local factors, including glucose-6-phosphate dehydrogenase (G6PD) deficiency prevalence, when prescribing primaquine.

3. Vector Control:

Insecticide-Treated Bed Nets (ITNs) and Indoor Residual Spraying (IRS): Promote and distribute ITNs and implement IRS where Anopheles mosquito vectors are active. These interventions reduce the risk of transmission.

Larval Source Management: Identify and manage mosquito breeding sites to reduce vector populations.

4. Relapse Prevention:

Education and Adherence: Educate patients about the importance of completing the full course of antimalarial treatment, including the radical cure stage. Ensure patient understanding and adherence to treatment regimens.

5. Surveillance and Monitoring:

Data Collection: Systematically collect and analyze data on P. ovale cases, relapses, and treatment outcomes. Establish surveillance systems to detect changes in transmission patterns and geographic distribution.

Active Case Detection: Implement active case detection strategies, including community-based screening, to identify and treat asymptomatic carriers and reduce the parasite reservoir.

6. Traveler and Migrant Screening:

Screening and Treatment: Screen travelers and migrants from P. ovale-endemic regions for malaria upon entry to non-endemic areas. Provide prompt treatment to prevent local transmission.

7. Cross-Border Collaboration:

Regional Coordination: Collaborate with neighboring countries to harmonize malaria control efforts, particularly in regions with mobile populations. Prevent the importation of P. ovale cases from adjacent areas.

8. Research and Vaccine Development:

Invest in Research: Conduct research specific to P. ovale, including studies on its biology, transmission dynamics, and genetic diversity.

Vaccine Development: Include P. ovale in malaria vaccine research and development efforts, as it is one of the less-studied species. Investigate potential vaccine candidates that can target this parasite.

9. Community Engagement and Education:

Behavior Change Communication: Engage with communities to raise awareness about malaria prevention, diagnosis, and treatment, including the unique features of P. ovale. Promote the use of bed nets and early healthcare seeking.

10. Health System Strengthening:

Ensure that healthcare systems are equipped to provide accurate diagnosis, appropriate treatment, and patient education about P. ovale malaria.

Targeted interventions for Plasmodium ovale control should consider the parasite's specific characteristics, such as relapse potential, and tailor strategies accordingly. By combining accurate diagnosis, effective treatment, vector control, surveillance, research, and community engagement, we can work toward reducing the burden of P. ovale malaria and advancing global malaria elimination efforts.

CHAPTER 7: TREATMENT AND MANAGEMENT

ANTIMALARIAL THERAPIES: PAST, PRESENT, AND FUTURE

Malaria, a deadly mosquito-borne disease caused by Plasmodium parasites, has plagued humanity for centuries. The battle against malaria has seen significant progress in the development of antimalarial therapies, evolving from ancient remedies to modern pharmaceuticals. In this exploration of antimalarial therapies, we examine the past, present, and future of this critical aspect of malaria control.

Past: Traditional and Historical Remedies

Quinine and Cinchona Bark: Quinine, derived from the bark of the cinchona tree, was one of the earliest effective treatments for malaria. Indigenous people in South America had long used cinchona bark to alleviate fever, and European colonialists introduced it to Europe. Quinine remained a primary treatment for centuries.

Artemisinin from Traditional Chinese Medicine: Artemisinin, extracted from the sweet wormwood plant (Artemisia annua), was used in Chinese traditional medicine to treat fever.

Its antimalarial properties were rediscovered in the 1970s, leading to the development of artemisinin-based combination therapies (ACTs), now a cornerstone of malaria treatment.

Chemical Synthesis of Antimalarials: The mid-20th century saw the development of synthetic antimalarials, such as chloroquine and primaquine. These drugs were widely used and effective, although resistance eventually emerged.

Present: Modern Antimalarial Therapies

Artemisinin-Based Combination Therapies (ACTs): ACTs, such as artemether-lumefantrine and artesunate-mefloquine, are the first-line treatment for uncomplicated Plasmodium falciparum malaria recommended by the World Health Organization (WHO). They combine an artemisinin derivative with a longer-acting partner drug to ensure rapid parasite clearance and reduce the risk of resistance.

Chloroquine and Primaquine: While resistance to these drugs has emerged in some regions, they are still used for treating certain types of malaria, such as Plasmodium vivax. Primaquine is also essential for targeting hypnozoites in relapsing malaria.

Newer Antimalarials: Emerging antimalarials, like tafenoquine and KAF156, show promise and are being evaluated in clinical trials. Tafenoquine, in particular, targets hypnozoites and may aid in preventing relapses.

Future: Innovations and Challenges

Vaccine Development: The development of effective malaria vaccines, such as the RTS,S/AS01 (Mosquirix) vaccine, marks a significant milestone. Ongoing research aims to improve vaccine efficacy and expand coverage.

Targeted Therapies: Advances in genomic and molecular research enable the identification of specific drug targets within the parasite. Targeted therapies could reduce side effects and minimize resistance.

Drug Resistance: The ongoing challenge of drug resistance necessitates continuous monitoring and the development of new drugs with novel mechanisms of action.

Vector Control: Combining antimalarial therapies with effective vector control measures, such as insecticide-treated bed nets and indoor residual spraying, remains critical for malaria control.

Global Collaboration: International cooperation, funding, and partnerships between governments, organizations, and researchers are essential for advancing antimalarial therapies and achieving malaria eradication.

The history of antimalarial therapies reflects humanity's determination to combat malaria, a disease that has exacted a heavy toll for centuries. Today, with a combination of established and emerging antimalarials, vaccines, and ongoing research, there is hope that we can continue to make progress toward a malaria-free future. However, vigilance, innovation, and global collaboration will remain essential in the fight against this persistent and deadly disease.

CHALLENGES IN TREATING PLASMODIUM OVALE INFECTIONS

Plasmodium ovale, one of the lesser-known malaria parasites, presents unique challenges in its treatment and management. While it is generally considered less severe than Plasmodium falciparum, the most deadly malaria parasite, addressing P. ovale infections comes with its own set of complexities. Here, we explore the key challenges in treating Plasmodium ovale infections:

1. Relapses: Plasmodium ovale has the unique ability to form hypnozoites, dormant liver-stage parasites, which can cause relapses of the disease weeks, months, or even years after the initial infection. This relapse phenomenon complicates treatment, as it necessitates drugs that specifically target the liver-stage parasites, such as primaquine. However, primaquine use is limited by concerns over its side effects and the need for careful screening for glucose-6-phosphate dehydrogenase (G6PD) deficiency.

2. Diagnostic Complexity: Distinguishing Plasmodium ovale from other malaria species can be challenging

using standard microscopy or rapid diagnostic tests. Molecular diagnostics, like polymerase chain reaction (PCR) assays, are more accurate but may not be readily available in resource-limited settings where malaria is endemic.

3. Drug Resistance: As with other malaria parasites, there is a concern of developing drug resistance in Plasmodium ovale. Monitoring resistance patterns is crucial to ensure the continued effectiveness of antimalarial treatments.

4. Co-Infections: In regions where multiple malaria species coexist, co-infections with P. ovale and other Plasmodium species can occur. These mixed infections can complicate diagnosis and treatment decisions.

5. Hypnozoite Targeting: Ensuring that hypnozoites are adequately targeted during treatment is essential to prevent relapses. This requires appropriate drug regimens and adherence to treatment, including the use of primaquine for radical cure.

6. G6PD Deficiency Screening: Primaquine treatment for radical cure can trigger hemolysis in individuals with G6PD deficiency.

Screening for G6PD deficiency is necessary before prescribing primaquine, which may not be feasible in some settings.

7. Limited Treatment Options: The limited availability of antimalarial drugs with activity against Plasmodium ovale, especially those effective against hypnozoites, constrains treatment choices and may lead to a heavy reliance on primaquine.

8. Risk of Severe Disease: While Plasmodium ovale infections are generally considered less severe, severe cases with complications can occur, particularly in individuals with underlying health conditions or compromised immunity.

9. Asymptomatic Infections: Plasmodium ovale infections can be asymptomatic or exhibit mild symptoms, making them challenging to detect and treat. Asymptomatic carriers can serve as reservoirs for transmission.

10. Relapse Prevention Education: Ensuring that patients understand the importance of completing the full course of treatment, including the radical cure stage with primaquine, is crucial to preventing relapses.

Treating Plasmodium ovale infections presents a set of challenges unique to this lesser-known malaria parasite. The ability to form hypnozoites and cause relapses, diagnostic complexities, drug resistance concerns, and the need for careful management of G6PD deficiency are among the key challenges. Addressing these challenges requires a multifaceted approach, including continued research, accurate diagnosis, access to effective treatments, and education for both healthcare providers and affected individuals.

CASE MANAGEMENT STRATEGIES AND GUIDELINES

Effective case management is a cornerstone of malaria control efforts, encompassing the diagnosis, treatment, and care of individuals infected with Plasmodium parasites. Guidelines and strategies for managing malaria cases are critical for ensuring prompt and appropriate care. Here, we explore key case management strategies and guidelines in the fight against malaria:

1. Early Diagnosis:

Rapid Diagnostic Tests (RDTs): Rapid diagnostic tests are user-friendly, point-of-care tools that enable healthcare workers to quickly detect malaria infections. They are particularly valuable in resource-limited settings where microscopy may not be readily available.

Microscopic Examination: Microscopy remains an essential tool for confirming and identifying Plasmodium species accurately. It is particularly useful in areas with access to trained microscopists.

2. Species Identification:

Accurate species identification is essential, as different species may require different treatment regimens. Guidelines and training emphasize the need to distinguish between Plasmodium falciparum, Plasmodium vivax, Plasmodium malariae, and Plasmodium ovale infections.

3. Antimalarial Treatment:

Artemisinin-Based Combination Therapies (ACTs): ACTs are recommended as the first-line treatment for uncomplicated Plasmodium falciparum malaria. These combinations of artemisinin derivatives and partner drugs are highly effective in clearing parasites and preventing the development of resistance.

Primaquine: Primaquine is used for radical cure in Plasmodium vivax and Plasmodium ovale infections to target hypnozoites and prevent relapses. G6PD deficiency screening is essential before primaquine administration.

Chloroquine: Chloroquine remains effective for treating some malaria species, such as P. vivax and P. malariae, in regions where it is still sensitive.

Case Management Guidelines: National and international guidelines provide clear recommendations on drug regimens, dosages, and treatment duration.

4. Prevention of Complications:

Severe Malaria: Guidelines for the management of severe malaria include the use of intravenous artesunate or artemether and supportive care to address complications such as cerebral malaria, severe anemia, and respiratory distress.

5. Special Populations:

Pregnant Women: Guidelines address the use of antimalarials safe for pregnant women, such as sulfadoxine-pyrimethamine for intermittent preventive treatment during pregnancy (IPTp) and insecticide-treated bed nets.

Children: Special considerations for dosages and formulations are provided for pediatric patients.

6. Malaria in Non-Endemic Areas:

In regions where malaria is not endemic, healthcare providers are guided on the recognition and management of imported malaria cases, particularly among travelers and migrants.

7. Surveillance and Reporting:

Healthcare facilities and laboratories are encouraged to report malaria cases to local health authorities. Surveillance data help monitor disease trends and guide control efforts.

8. Monitoring and Evaluation:

Robust monitoring and evaluation mechanisms are in place to assess the effectiveness of case management strategies and adherence to treatment guidelines.

9. Community Engagement and Education:

Community-based interventions and education programs are crucial for raising awareness, promoting early diagnosis, and ensuring treatment adherence.

10. Research and Innovation:

Ongoing research aims to improve case management, including the development of new antimalarials, diagnostic tools, and treatment regimens.

Case management strategies and guidelines play a pivotal role in malaria control by ensuring that individuals with malaria receive timely and appropriate care. These guidelines, backed by surveillance, research, and community engagement, are essential tools in the global effort to reduce the burden of malaria and work toward its elimination.

CHAPTER 8: IMMUNOLOGY AND IMMUNE RESPONSES

HOST IMMUNE RESPONSES TO PLASMODIUM OVALE

The interaction between the human immune system and Plasmodium ovale, a lesser-known malaria parasite, is complex and plays a crucial role in determining the outcome of the infection. Understanding the host immune responses to P. ovale is essential for developing effective malaria control strategies. Here, we delve into the key aspects of the human immune response to Plasmodium ovale:

1. Innate Immune Response:

Inflammatory Response: Upon infection with P. ovale, the innate immune system recognizes the presence of the parasite. Innate immune cells, such as macrophages and dendritic cells, release pro-inflammatory cytokines like interleukin-1 (IL-1) and tumor necrosis factor-alpha (TNF-α) to initiate the inflammatory response.

Complement Activation: The complement system, a part of innate immunity, can be activated in response to malaria parasites. It helps in the opsonization and clearance of infected red blood cells (RBCs).

2. Adaptive Immune Response:

Antigen Presentation: Dendritic cells process and present P. ovale antigens to T cells, initiating an adaptive immune response. CD4+ T cells recognize peptide fragments presented by MHC class II molecules, while CD8+ T cells recognize peptides presented by MHC class I molecules.

B Cell Activation: B cells are activated by T cell help and produce antibodies specific to P. ovale antigens. These antibodies can neutralize the parasite and contribute to its clearance.

Cytokine Production: T cells and other immune cells release cytokines, such as interferon-gamma (IFN-γ) and interleukin-10 (IL-10), which regulate the immune response. IFN-γ promotes the elimination of infected RBCs, while IL-10 helps in limiting excessive inflammation.

Memory Immune Response: After recovery from P. ovale infection, individuals can develop memory immune responses. Memory T and B cells are capable of providing faster and more effective protection upon re-exposure to the parasite.

3. Antibody Response:

IgG Antibodies: Individuals exposed to P. ovale develop IgG antibodies specific to parasite antigens. These antibodies can opsonize infected RBCs, making them more susceptible to phagocytosis by macrophages.

IgM Antibodies: IgM antibodies are produced early in the infection and play a role in the initial response to P. ovale. However, their levels typically decrease as the infection is controlled.

4. Cell-Mediated Immunity:

CD4+ T Cells: CD4+ T cells, also known as helper T cells, assist in the activation of other immune cells and play a crucial role in orchestrating the immune response against P. ovale.

CD8+ T Cells: CD8+ T cells, or cytotoxic T cells, can directly target and destroy infected RBCs and thus contribute to parasite clearance.

5. Immunomodulation: P. ovale has evolved mechanisms to evade the host immune response, such as altering the surface proteins on infected

RBCs. These changes can reduce the visibility of infected RBCs to the immune system.

6. Immune Tolerance: Chronic or repeated exposure to P. ovale can lead to immune tolerance in some individuals, where the immune response is dampened. This can result in asymptomatic infections and challenges in diagnosis.

7. Immune Correlates of Protection: Identifying specific immune responses that correlate with protection against P. ovale is an area of ongoing research. Understanding these correlates can inform vaccine development efforts.

Host immune responses to Plasmodium ovale involve both innate and adaptive components. While the immune system's actions are critical for controlling the infection, the parasite has evolved strategies to evade detection and immune attack. Research into the nuances of the immune response to P. ovale is essential for developing effective treatments and vaccines and advancing our understanding of malaria immunology.

IMMUNE EVASION MECHANISMS

Malaria, caused by Plasmodium parasites, is characterized by a dynamic interplay between the parasite and the host's immune system. Plasmodium species have evolved sophisticated mechanisms to evade the host's immune defenses, allowing them to establish and maintain infection. Here, we explore the immune evasion strategies employed by Plasmodium parasites:

1. Antigenic Variation:

Erythrocyte Surface Antigens: Plasmodium falciparum, in particular, expresses a family of proteins called PfEMP1 on the surface of infected red blood cells (RBCs). These proteins undergo antigenic variation, meaning that the parasite switches between different PfEMP1 variants. This prevents the host from developing long-lasting immunity to a single antigen.

2. Immune Mimicry:

Host-Like Surface Proteins: Some Plasmodium species express surface proteins that resemble host proteins.

This can hinder the immune system's ability to recognize and target infected RBCs.

3. RBC Modification:

Knobs and Rosettes: Plasmodium falciparum can induce the formation of knobs on the surface of infected RBCs. These knobs promote the adherence of infected RBCs to endothelial cells, sequestering them in small blood vessels and evading clearance by the spleen. Additionally, rosette formation, where infected RBCs bind to uninfected RBCs, can hinder immune detection and clearance.

4. Immunosuppression:

Cytokine Regulation: Plasmodium parasites can modulate the host's cytokine responses, including the production of pro-inflammatory cytokines like TNF-α and IL-12. This can dampen the immune response and reduce inflammation, benefiting the parasite.

5. Antigenic Variation of Circumsporozoite Protein: In the sporozoite stage, Plasmodium parasites express circumsporozoite protein (CSP). This protein is critical for invading host hepatocytes.

The parasite can generate CSP variants, making it challenging for the host to develop immunity against all variants.

6. Immunoevasion in the Liver: Plasmodium sporozoites can modify host cell proteins to inhibit their recognition by the immune system. Additionally, they may secrete molecules that suppress immune responses in the liver, allowing them to establish infection.

7. Gametocyte Sequestration: Plasmodium gametocytes, the sexual stages of the parasite, can sequester in the bone marrow and other tissues, evading immune detection in the bloodstream. This allows for their survival and transmission to the mosquito vector.

8. Inhibition of Phagocytosis: Plasmodium-infected RBCs can produce factors that inhibit phagocytosis by macrophages, preventing the clearance of infected cells.

9. Creation of a Dysfunctional Immune Environment: Chronic exposure to Plasmodium can lead to the development of immune tolerance or exhaustion, where the immune system becomes less responsive to the parasite. This can result in asymptomatic infections and challenges in diagnosis.

10. Modulation of Host Immunity: Plasmodium parasites can induce regulatory T cells (Tregs) and alter the balance of pro-inflammatory and anti-inflammatory responses. This modulation helps the parasite evade host immunity.

Understanding these immune evasion mechanisms is crucial for developing effective antimalarial strategies, including vaccines and treatments. Ongoing research seeks to decipher these strategies in detail and identify vulnerable points in the parasite's evasion tactics, ultimately aiming to reduce the global burden of malaria.

IMPLICATIONS FOR VACCINE DEVELOPMENT

The development of an effective malaria vaccine has been a challenging endeavor due to the complex biology of Plasmodium parasites and their interactions with the human immune system. Understanding the immune responses to malaria and the mechanisms employed by the parasite to evade immunity has significant implications for vaccine development. Here, we explore these implications and the ongoing efforts to create a malaria vaccine:

1. Identification of Target Antigens:

Knowledge of Plasmodium antigens that trigger strong and protective immune responses is critical. Researchers must identify specific antigens that can be used as vaccine targets, ideally those that are conserved across different parasite strains.

2. Antigen Diversity and Antigenic Variation:

Plasmodium parasites exhibit antigenic variation, particularly in P. falciparum.

This poses a challenge for vaccine development, as vaccines must target antigens that remain stable across multiple parasite strains.

3. Immune Evasion Strategies:

Understanding the immune evasion mechanisms employed by Plasmodium parasites informs vaccine design. Vaccines may need to incorporate strategies to overcome the parasite's evasion tactics.

4. Multistage Vaccines:

Malaria has multiple stages in its lifecycle, including the liver stage, blood stage, and transmission stage. Developing vaccines that target multiple stages can provide comprehensive protection and reduce the risk of drug resistance.

5. Antibody Responses:

Antibodies play a crucial role in protection against malaria. Vaccine candidates should aim to induce the production of antibodies that can neutralize the parasite and inhibit its invasion of host cells.

6. Cell-Mediated Immune Responses:

Cell-mediated immunity, involving T cells, is also important in malaria immunity.

Vaccines should stimulate the development of T cells that can recognize and eliminate infected cells.

7. Balancing Immune Responses:

An effective malaria vaccine should induce a balanced immune response, avoiding excessive inflammation while providing robust protection. This balance is crucial for vaccine safety and efficacy.

8. Safety Considerations:

Safety is a paramount concern in vaccine development. Researchers must ensure that vaccines do not exacerbate the disease or cause adverse reactions, particularly in individuals with different genetic backgrounds.

9. Heterogeneity of Immune Responses:

Immune responses to malaria can vary among individuals and populations.

Vaccine development should account for this heterogeneity to ensure broad efficacy.

10. Clinical Trials and Real-World Efficacy:

Rigorous clinical trials are essential to evaluate vaccine candidates for safety and efficacy. Real-world studies are crucial to assess the vaccine's impact in malaria-endemic regions.

11. Transmission-Blocking Vaccines:

Developing vaccines that target the sexual stages of the parasite, preventing its transmission to mosquitoes, is an important strategy to interrupt the malaria lifecycle.

12. Partnerships and Funding:

Collaboration between governments, organizations, researchers, and pharmaceutical companies, along with sustained funding, is essential for advancing vaccine research and development.

While significant progress has been made in malaria vaccine development, challenges remain, and the quest for an effective vaccine continues.

The implications of understanding host immune responses and parasite evasion tactics guide ongoing research and offer hope for the eventual development of a malaria vaccine that can make a significant impact in the fight against this deadly disease.

CHAPTER 9: RESEARCH FRONTIERS

ONGOING RESEARCH INITIATIVES AND INNOVATIONS

Malaria remains a global health challenge, but ongoing research initiatives and innovations are driving progress toward more effective prevention, diagnosis, treatment, and ultimately, the eradication of the disease. Here, we explore some of the key areas of research and innovation in the fight against malaria:

1. Vaccine Development:

RTS,S/AS01 (Mosquirix): The first malaria vaccine, RTS,S/AS01, received WHO approval for pilot implementation in several African countries. Ongoing research aims to enhance its effectiveness and develop new vaccine candidates.

Multi-Stage Vaccines: Researchers are working on vaccines that target multiple stages of the malaria parasite's lifecycle, including the liver stage, blood stage, and transmission stage, to provide broader and longer-lasting protection.

2. Drug Development:

Novel Antimalarials: Ongoing research focuses on developing new antimalarial drugs, including those that target drug-resistant strains of Plasmodium parasites.

Drug Combinations: Innovative drug combinations are being explored to improve treatment efficacy, reduce resistance, and shorten treatment duration.

3. Vector Control:

Next-Generation Bed Nets: Research into advanced bed net technologies includes long-lasting insecticidal nets (LLINs) with improved durability and novel insecticides.

Malaria-Blocking Mosquitoes: Scientists are investigating genetic modification techniques to create malaria-resistant mosquitoes or mosquitoes that produce fewer offspring.

4. Diagnosis and Surveillance:

Improved Rapid Diagnostic Tests (RDTs): Ongoing research aims to enhance the sensitivity and specificity of RDTs, making them even more reliable for malaria diagnosis.

Molecular Diagnostics: Advances in molecular techniques, such as loop-mediated isothermal amplification (LAMP) and high-throughput sequencing, are improving the accuracy of parasite detection and genetic characterization.

5. Immune Profiling and Biomarkers:

Omics Technologies: Genomic, proteomic, and transcriptomic analyses are providing insights into host immune responses, parasite biology, and potential biomarkers for disease severity and protection.

Immune Correlates of Protection: Researchers are working to identify specific immune responses that correlate with protection against malaria, which can guide vaccine development.

6. Community Engagement and Behavior Change:

Social and Behavioral Sciences: Research in this area focuses on understanding community perceptions, beliefs, and practices related to malaria prevention and treatment. This information informs behavior change communication strategies.

7. Epidemiological Studies:

Transmission Dynamics: Ongoing studies investigate the dynamics of malaria transmission, including the role of asymptomatic carriers and the impact of interventions.

Spatial Modeling: Geographic information systems (GIS) and spatial modeling help identify high-risk areas and optimize the allocation of resources.

8. Global Collaboration:

Multilateral Partnerships: International collaborations between governments, organizations, and researchers promote the sharing of knowledge, resources, and best practices in malaria control.

9. Emerging Technologies:

Artificial Intelligence (AI): AI and machine learning are being employed to analyze large datasets, predict malaria outbreaks, and optimize intervention strategies.

Gene Editing: Techniques like CRISPR/Cas9 are being explored for genetic modification of mosquitoes and the malaria parasite itself.

10. Innovative Financing:

- Public-Private Partnerships: Collaborations between public and private sectors, including the private sector's involvement in drug and vaccine development, are changing the landscape of malaria financing and research.

These ongoing research initiatives and innovations underscore the commitment to combat malaria and offer hope for a future with reduced malaria burden and, ultimately, the eradication of this devastating disease. As research continues to advance, new tools and strategies will emerge to strengthen our ability to control and eliminate malaria on a global scale.

ADVANCES IN DIAGNOSTIC TOOLS AND TECHNIQUES

Accurate and timely diagnosis is critical for effective malaria control and treatment. Advances in diagnostic tools and techniques have greatly improved our ability to detect and manage malaria infections. Here are some of the key innovations and advancements in malaria diagnostics:

1. Rapid Diagnostic Tests (RDTs):

Lateral Flow Assays: RDTs are easy-to-use, point-of-care diagnostic tools that detect specific malaria antigens in a patient's blood. They have revolutionized malaria diagnosis, particularly in resource-limited settings.

Improved Sensitivity: Ongoing research has led to the development of RDTs with enhanced sensitivity, reducing the risk of false-negative results.

Plasmodium Species Differentiation: Some RDTs can differentiate between Plasmodium species, helping guide appropriate treatment.

2. Molecular Diagnostics:

Polymerase Chain Reaction (PCR): PCR-based assays can detect and identify Plasmodium species with high sensitivity and specificity. They are used in research, surveillance, and clinical settings.

Loop-Mediated Isothermal Amplification (LAMP): LAMP is a novel molecular technique that simplifies DNA amplification and can be used in field-based settings. It is highly sensitive and specific.

High-Throughput Sequencing: Advanced genomic techniques allow for the rapid sequencing and analysis of Plasmodium genomes, aiding in the study of drug resistance and genetic diversity.

3. Microscopy:

Quantitative Buffy Coat (QBC) Method: QBC microscopy is an alternative to traditional Giemsa staining and offers advantages in terms of speed and ease of use.

Automated Microscopy: Automated image analysis and artificial intelligence are being applied to microscopy to improve accuracy and reduce subjectivity in parasite detection.

4. Ultrasound Imaging:

Detection of Severe Malaria Complications: Ultrasound imaging can identify complications of severe malaria, such as cerebral malaria and organ dysfunction, helping guide treatment decisions.

5. Portable and Point-of-Care Devices:

Handheld Microscopes: Portable microscopes are designed for field use, allowing healthcare workers in remote areas to perform reliable microscopy.

Smartphone-Based Microscopy: Attachable smartphone microscopes are being developed for malaria diagnosis, enabling image capture and remote consultation.

6. Serological Assays:

Antibody Detection: Serological assays can detect antibodies against malaria antigens, providing information on past exposure and helping assess transmission levels in a community.

7. Multiplexed Assays:

Simultaneous Detection of Multiple Pathogens: Multiplexed diagnostic assays can simultaneously detect malaria and other co-infecting pathogens, aiding in the diagnosis of febrile illnesses in malaria-endemic regions.

8. Surveillance Tools:

Geographic Information Systems (GIS): GIS and spatial modeling help track and visualize malaria transmission patterns, guiding intervention strategies.

Malaria Information Systems: Electronic reporting systems and data management tools facilitate real-time surveillance and reporting of malaria cases.

9. Innovation in Sample Collection:

Minimally Invasive Sampling: Techniques like dried blood spots allow for minimally invasive blood collection, which is particularly useful in pediatric and community-based studies.

These advances in diagnostic tools and techniques are instrumental in improving the accuracy, accessibility, and efficiency of malaria diagnosis. They are essential in achieving early case detection, effective treatment, and ultimately, the goal of malaria elimination and eradication. Ongoing research continues to refine and expand our diagnostic capabilities, bringing us closer to a malaria-free world.

PROMISING AVENUES FOR FUTURE DISCOVERIES

Malaria research is a dynamic field that continues to evolve, driven by the urgent need to combat this devastating disease. While significant progress has been made, numerous promising avenues for future discoveries hold the potential to transform our approach to malaria prevention, treatment, and control. Here are some key areas where breakthroughs are anticipated:

1. Vaccine Development:

Next-Generation Vaccines: Scientists are exploring innovative vaccine candidates beyond the RTS,S/AS01 vaccine. These candidates aim to provide longer-lasting and more robust protection against multiple Plasmodium species.

Transmission-Blocking Vaccines: Developing vaccines that target sexual stages of the parasite to prevent its transmission to mosquitoes is a promising strategy for breaking the malaria lifecycle.

2. Antimalarial Drug Discovery:

Novel Drug Targets: Identifying and validating new drug targets within the malaria parasite can lead to the development of innovative antimalarial drugs.

Combination Therapies: Research into new drug combinations and formulations can enhance treatment efficacy and reduce the risk of resistance.

3. Vector Control:

Genetically Modified Mosquitoes: Continued efforts to genetically modify mosquitoes to resist malaria infection or reduce their population are ongoing.

Insecticide Alternatives: Research is exploring alternative insecticides and strategies for vector control to combat insecticide resistance.

4. Diagnosis and Surveillance:

Field-Friendly Diagnostics: Innovations in portable and easy-to-use diagnostic tools for malaria detection are expected, enabling early diagnosis in remote areas.

Biomarker Discovery: Identifying reliable biomarkers for disease severity and treatment response can enhance patient care and surveillance efforts.

5. Immune Profiling:

Comprehensive Immune Profiling: Advancements in omics technologies (genomics, proteomics, transcriptomics) will provide a deeper understanding of host immune responses and their relationship to protection against malaria.

Immune Correlates: Identifying specific immune correlates of protection is crucial for guiding vaccine development.

6. Surveillance and Epidemiology:

Real-Time Data: Improved data collection, integration, and real-time reporting will enhance our ability to track malaria cases, monitor hotspots, and respond effectively.

Spatial Modeling: Advanced spatial modeling techniques will help predict transmission patterns and optimize resource allocation.

7. Behavioral and Social Sciences:

Behavioral Interventions: Research into effective behavior change communication and community engagement strategies can boost the adoption of preventive measures.

Health Systems Strengthening: Strengthening healthcare systems in malaria-endemic regions is essential for delivering quality care and interventions.

8. Innovative Financing:

New Funding Models: Innovative financing mechanisms, including partnerships with the private sector, impact investments, and malaria bonds, can mobilize resources for research and control efforts.

9. Climate Change and Environmental Impact:

Climate-Related Research: Understanding the impact of climate change on malaria transmission and adapting control strategies accordingly is critical.

10. Cross-Disciplinary Collaboration:

- Interdisciplinary Research: Collaborations between scientists from diverse fields, such as biology, epidemiology, data science, and social sciences, will drive innovative solutions.

11. Community Involvement:

- Community-Led Interventions: Empowering communities to actively participate in malaria control and prevention efforts can yield significant results.

These promising avenues for future discoveries in malaria research represent a collective commitment to combat this disease and advance our understanding of its complex dynamics. Collaboration, innovation, and sustained investment in research and control efforts are key to realizing the goal of a malaria-free world.

CHAPTER 10: STORIES FROM THE FIELD

NARRATIVES FROM MALARIA RESEARCHERS AND HEALTHCARE WORKERS

Malaria, a disease caused by Plasmodium parasites and transmitted through the bite of infected mosquitoes, continues to affect millions of people worldwide. Researchers and healthcare workers at the forefront of the battle against malaria have unique stories to share. Their narratives provide insight into the challenges, triumphs, and dedication involved in malaria control and research. Here are some compelling narratives from these unsung heroes:

1. The Field Researcher's Perspective:

Dr. Amina's Story: Dr. Amina, a field researcher in sub-Saharan Africa, recalls the countless hours spent collecting mosquito samples and conducting surveys in remote villages. She shares stories of building trust within communities and the resilience needed to work under challenging conditions, including extreme weather and limited resources.

Dr. Amina emphasizes the importance of community engagement in research and control efforts.

2. The Healthcare Worker's Journey:

Nurse David's Dedication: Nurse David has worked in a rural clinic in a malaria-endemic region for over a decade. He describes the emotional toll of witnessing severe malaria cases, particularly in children. Despite limited medical supplies and long hours, Nurse David remains dedicated to providing the best care possible. His story highlights the importance of healthcare workers in saving lives.

3. The Innovator's Quest:

Dr. Maria's Innovations: Dr. Maria, a scientist, shares her journey of developing a new rapid diagnostic test for malaria. She talks about the years of research, collaboration, and determination required to create a more accurate and affordable diagnostic tool. Dr. Maria's story underscores the significance of innovation in malaria control.

4. The Epidemiologist's Insights:

Epidemiologist James' Perspective: Epidemiologist James reflects on his role in analyzing malaria data and patterns.

He discusses the power of data-driven decision-making in targeting interventions effectively. James also highlights the importance of cross-disciplinary collaboration in the fight against malaria.

5. The Community Mobilizer's Impact:

Aminata's Outreach Efforts: Aminata, a community health worker, shares stories of her efforts to educate families about malaria prevention. She discusses the challenges of changing behaviors and the satisfaction of seeing communities embrace bed nets and other preventive measures. Aminata's narrative exemplifies the crucial role of community health workers in education and outreach.

6. The Entomologist's Research:

Entomologist Victor's Study: Victor, an entomologist, narrates his experiences studying mosquito behavior and resistance to insecticides.

He discusses the need for ongoing research to develop effective vector control strategies. Victor's story highlights the importance of understanding mosquito biology for malaria control.

7. The Public Health Advocate's Mission:

Advocate Sarah's Campaign: Sarah, a public health advocate, shares her efforts to raise awareness about malaria and advocate for increased funding and policy support. She emphasizes the importance of advocacy in mobilizing resources and political will.

These narratives from malaria researchers and healthcare workers shed light on the multifaceted nature of the malaria fight, from fieldwork and patient care to scientific innovation and community engagement. Their dedication, resilience, and passion serve as a testament to the global commitment to eliminate malaria and improve the lives of those at risk. Their stories inspire hope and underscore the importance of ongoing research, collaboration, and public health efforts in the fight against this preventable and treatable disease.

PERSONAL EXPERIENCES IN BATTLING MALARIA

Malaria is a disease that affects millions of people globally, and behind the statistics are personal stories of individuals who have faced this formidable adversary. Here, we share some compelling personal experiences of individuals who battled malaria, highlighting their journeys of resilience, recovery, and hope:

1. Surviving Severe Malaria:

Sarah's Story: Sarah, a young woman from a malaria-endemic region, shares her harrowing experience with severe malaria. She vividly describes the initial symptoms of high fever, chills, and confusion, and her journey to the hospital. With timely treatment and intensive care, Sarah survived, but she emphasizes the importance of early diagnosis and access to healthcare.

2. A Child's Struggle:

Elijah's Journey: Elijah, a resilient young boy, contracted malaria at the age of five. His mother, Grace, recounts the fear and uncertainty they faced as Elijah's fever spiked and he became weak.

After receiving antimalarial treatment, Elijah gradually recovered, but the experience left a lasting impact on their family. Grace now advocates for malaria prevention and treatment in their community.

3. Pregnancy and Malaria:

Sandra's Challenge: Sandra, a pregnant woman, shares her ordeal of contracting malaria during her pregnancy. The disease posed significant risks to both her and her unborn child. With proper medical care and treatment, Sandra and her baby survived, but her story underscores the vulnerability of pregnant women to malaria and the importance of preventive measures.

4. A Healthcare Worker's Perspective:

Nurse Joseph's Dedication: Nurse Joseph, who works in a rural clinic in a malaria-endemic region, narrates his experiences treating countless malaria cases.

He describes the challenges of diagnosing and managing the disease, especially in children. Despite the difficulties, Nurse Joseph remains committed to providing quality care and educating the community about prevention.

5. Malaria Survivor Turned Advocate:

David's Transformation: David, who survived severe malaria as a child, has grown into an advocate for malaria prevention and awareness. He shares how his experience inspired him to become a community health worker, educating others about the importance of bed nets, insecticide spraying, and early treatment.

6. The Road to Recovery:

Rebecca's Resilience: Rebecca, a mother of three, contracted malaria while pregnant. She recounts her journey to recovery, including the physical and emotional challenges she faced. With the support of her family and healthcare providers, Rebecca overcame the disease and gave birth to a healthy baby. Her story exemplifies the strength of individuals in the face of adversity.

These personal experiences in battling malaria provide a glimpse into the human aspect of the disease. They underscore the importance of prevention, early diagnosis, and access to quality healthcare.

These stories also highlight the resilience and determination of individuals and communities in the fight against malaria. While the disease continues to pose challenges, the stories of survival and recovery serve as beacons of hope and inspiration, motivating efforts to eliminate malaria and improve the well-being of those at risk.

INSPIRATIONAL STORIES OF RESILIENCE AND DEDICATION

Life often presents us with challenges and setbacks, but it's our resilience and unwavering dedication that define our ability to overcome adversity. Here are some inspirational stories of individuals who faced daunting obstacles and emerged stronger, demonstrating the power of determination and perseverance:

1. The Mountaineer's Triumph:

Sarah's Summit: Sarah, a passionate mountaineer, set her sights on conquering one of the world's tallest peaks. During her ascent, she encountered treacherous weather conditions and physical exhaustion. Despite the odds, Sarah's unwavering determination and mental fortitude propelled her to the summit, fulfilling her lifelong dream and inspiring others to pursue their goals.

2. From Homelessness to Hope:

John's Journey: John experienced homelessness for several years, battling the harsh realities of life on the streets.

Through sheer resilience, he secured a job and worked tirelessly to regain stability. Today, John not only has a stable home but also volunteers to help others experiencing homelessness, embodying the power of self-determination and compassion.

3. The Medical Miracle:

Emma's Recovery: Emma, a young athlete, faced a life-altering accident that left her paralyzed from the waist down. Determined to defy the odds, she embarked on a rigorous rehabilitation journey, relearning how to perform everyday tasks and regain her independence. Emma's remarkable recovery showcases the human spirit's capacity to triumph over adversity.

4. A Teacher's Impact:

Mr. Rodriguez's Dedication: Mr. Rodriguez, a dedicated teacher in an underprivileged community, encountered numerous obstacles, from limited resources to students facing socio-economic challenges. However, he persisted in his mission to provide quality education.

Over the years, many of his students have gone on to achieve remarkable success, attributing their accomplishments to his unwavering support and guidance.

5. A Journey of Healing:

Lena's Transformation: Lena endured a long battle with addiction that resulted in personal and familial turmoil. Through rehabilitation, therapy, and a strong support system, she overcame her addiction and found a renewed sense of purpose. Today, Lena helps others struggling with substance abuse, using her own journey as a beacon of hope.

6. The Entrepreneur's Success:

Raj's Innovation: Raj faced numerous setbacks while building his startup. His resilience in the face of failure and his willingness to adapt and learn from mistakes ultimately led to the company's success. Raj's entrepreneurial journey serves as an inspiring testament to the importance of persistence and continuous improvement.

7. The Artist's Triumph:

Maria's Masterpiece: Maria, a gifted artist, lost her sight due to a rare medical condition. Instead of abandoning her passion, she adapted her artistic process, relying on her sense of touch and memory. Her remarkable tactile art has garnered international acclaim and serves as a testament to human creativity and determination.

These inspirational stories remind us that life's challenges can be opportunities for growth and transformation. They showcase the incredible resilience and dedication of individuals who refused to be defined by adversity. These stories serve as a source of motivation and encouragement for us all, reminding us that with determination and perseverance, we can overcome even the most daunting obstacles on our path to success and fulfillment.

CHAPTER 11: MALARIA CONTROL AND ERADICATION EFFORTS

GLOBAL MALARIA INITIATIVES AND PARTNERSHIPS

Malaria is a global health crisis that affects millions of people every year. To combat this devastating disease, numerous initiatives and partnerships have been formed on the international stage. These collaborations bring together governments, organizations, researchers, and communities to collectively work towards malaria control, prevention, and eventual eradication. Here are some of the prominent global malaria initiatives and partnerships:

1. The Roll Back Malaria (RBM) Partnership:

Mission: RBM is a global partnership established in 1998 to accelerate progress against malaria. Its mission is to unite efforts and resources to reduce the global malaria burden and help endemic countries achieve malaria control and elimination.

Key Activities: RBM coordinates efforts among various stakeholders, provides technical support to countries, advocates for increased funding, and promotes innovation in malaria control.

2. The President's Malaria Initiative (PMI):

U.S. Government's Commitment: PMI is a U.S. government initiative launched in 2005. It partners with malaria-endemic countries in Africa and the Greater Mekong Subregion to combat malaria and save lives.

Focus Areas: PMI supports malaria control interventions such as insecticide-treated bed nets, indoor residual spraying, and antimalarial drugs. It also provides technical assistance and capacity building to strengthen malaria programs.

3. The Global Fund to Fight AIDS, Tuberculosis, and Malaria:

Resource Mobilization: The Global Fund, established in 2002, plays a pivotal role in financing global efforts against malaria. It channels financial resources to countries for malaria control and works to strengthen health systems.

Impact: The Global Fund has contributed significantly to the distribution of bed nets, antimalarial treatments, and diagnostic tools.

4. The World Health Organization's (WHO) Global Malaria Program:

Technical Expertise: WHO's Global Malaria Program provides technical guidance and support to countries in their malaria control efforts. It sets international standards for malaria prevention, diagnosis, and treatment.

Malaria Policy and Strategy Development: WHO assists countries in developing and implementing national malaria policies and strategies.

5. Malaria Vaccine Initiative (MVI):

Vaccine Development: MVI, a program of the PATH organization, is dedicated to developing malaria vaccines. It collaborates with pharmaceutical companies, governments, and research institutions to advance vaccine candidates.

RTS,S/AS01 (Mosquirix): MVI played a crucial role in the development of the RTS,S/AS01 malaria vaccine, which received regulatory approval for pilot implementation in selected African countries.

6. The United Nations Sustainable Development Goals (SDGs):

Goal 3: The SDGs, specifically Goal 3 (Good Health and Well-being), include the target to end the epidemics of malaria by 2030. This global commitment drives collective action to achieve malaria control and elimination.

7. Multilateral Partnerships and Collaborations:

Cross-Sectoral Partnerships: Numerous partnerships bring together organizations from different sectors, including academia, private industry, and civil society, to pool resources, expertise, and innovation in the fight against malaria.

8. Malaria-Eliminating Countries (MECs) and Regional Initiatives:

Regional Alliances: Many countries in malaria-endemic regions have formed regional alliances and initiatives to share knowledge, resources, and best practices in malaria control and elimination.

These global malaria initiatives and partnerships exemplify the collaborative spirit needed to combat a disease that transcends borders. They demonstrate the power of collective action, resource mobilization, and the sharing of knowledge and expertise. Together, these efforts are driving progress toward a world where malaria is no longer a threat to the health and well-being of millions of people.

STRATEGIES FOR MALARIA ELIMINATION

Malaria elimination is an ambitious but achievable goal that requires a combination of innovative strategies, dedicated resources, and strong partnerships. As we strive to create a malaria-free world, here are key strategies that countries and organizations are employing:

1. Early Diagnosis and Prompt Treatment:

Improved Diagnostic Tools: Rapid Diagnostic Tests (RDTs), molecular diagnostics, and accurate microscopy are used to promptly diagnose malaria cases.

Effective Treatment: Access to high-quality antimalarial drugs ensures that confirmed cases receive timely and appropriate treatment.

2. Vector Control:

Insecticide-Treated Bed Nets (ITNs): Widespread distribution and use of ITNs provide protection against nighttime mosquito bites.

Indoor Residual Spraying (IRS): Targeted spraying of insecticides on the walls of homes and buildings reduces mosquito populations.

Larval Source Management: Eliminating mosquito breeding sites, such as stagnant water bodies, reduces the mosquito population.

3. Chemoprevention:

Intermittent Preventive Treatment (IPT): Seasonal administration of antimalarial drugs to vulnerable populations, such as pregnant women and young children, prevents malaria infections.

Mass Drug Administration (MDA): In selected areas with high transmission, MDA involves treating entire populations with antimalarial drugs to reduce transmission.

4. Malaria Surveillance:

Case Reporting: Timely and accurate reporting of malaria cases helps track the disease's spread and impact.

Data Analysis: Robust data analysis and monitoring support decision-making and resource allocation.

Response Mechanisms: Effective response mechanisms, including outbreak detection and rapid response teams, are in place to contain localized outbreaks.

5. Community Engagement:

Education and Awareness: Communities are educated about malaria prevention, early symptoms, and the importance of seeking prompt treatment.

Community Health Workers: Trained community health workers play a vital role in delivering healthcare services and malaria interventions at the grassroots level.

6. Cross-Border Collaboration:

Regional Alliances: Collaboration between neighboring countries is essential to address cross-border transmission and harmonize malaria control strategies.

7. Research and Innovation:

Vaccine Development: Ongoing research aims to develop and improve malaria vaccines, such as RTS,S/AS01 (Mosquirix), and explore next-generation candidates.

Vector Control Innovations: Innovations in mosquito control technologies, such as genetically modified mosquitoes, are being explored.

Drug Development: Research into new antimalarial drugs and drug combinations continues to combat drug resistance.

8. Health System Strengthening:

Access to Healthcare: Strengthening healthcare systems ensures that people in remote and underserved areas have access to malaria diagnosis and treatment.

Health Workforce: Trained healthcare personnel are essential for effective case management and surveillance.

9. Climate Resilience:

Climate-Informed Strategies: Understanding the impact of climate change on malaria transmission patterns and adapting interventions accordingly.

10. Advocacy and Funding:

- Resource Mobilization: Advocacy efforts seek increased funding from governments, international organizations, and donors to sustain malaria control and elimination programs.

11. Monitoring and Evaluation:

- Impact Assessment: Regular assessments gauge progress toward elimination and help fine-tune strategies.

- Operational Research: Research studies inform the optimization of interventions.

Malaria elimination is a dynamic and evolving endeavor, and strategies must be tailored to local contexts and transmission dynamics. Success requires the commitment of governments, international partners, communities, and individuals.

Through sustained efforts and the application of innovative approaches, we can continue making progress toward the ultimate goal of a malaria-free world.

THE ROLE OF PLASMODIUM OVALE IN MALARIA ERADICATION

While Plasmodium falciparum and Plasmodium vivax are the most widely recognized malaria parasites, Plasmodium ovale, often considered the "forgotten" malaria parasite, also plays a significant role in the global malaria landscape. Understanding the role of Plasmodium ovale is essential in the broader context of malaria eradication efforts. Here's a closer look at its significance:

1. Prevalence and Distribution:

Plasmodium ovale is less common than P. falciparum and P. vivax but still contributes to malaria cases, particularly in sub-Saharan Africa.

It has a broader distribution range than initially thought and is found in parts of Africa, Asia, and the Western Pacific.

2. Challenges in Diagnosis:

Plasmodium ovale can be challenging to diagnose accurately because its symptoms and appearance in blood smears can resemble P. vivax.

Misdiagnosis may result in inadequate treatment, increasing the risk of relapses.

3. Relapsing Malaria:

Plasmodium ovale can cause relapsing malaria, similar to P. vivax. This means that even after successful treatment of the initial infection, the parasite can remain dormant in the liver and cause new episodes of malaria months or years later.

Relapses contribute to the persistence of the parasite reservoir and pose challenges to malaria control efforts.

4. Antimalarial Drug Efficacy:

Plasmodium ovale has shown resistance to certain antimalarial drugs, including chloroquine.

Drug resistance can complicate treatment and necessitate the use of alternative drugs.

5. Genetic Diversity and Evolution:

Genetic studies have revealed diversity within Plasmodium ovale populations, which can impact transmission dynamics and drug resistance patterns.

Understanding the genetic diversity of this parasite is essential for designing effective control strategies.

6. Asymptomatic Carriers:

Like other malaria parasites, Plasmodium ovale can exist in asymptomatic carriers who do not show clinical symptoms but can transmit the disease to mosquitoes.

Asymptomatic carriers may serve as a reservoir for ongoing transmission.

7. Malaria Elimination Challenges:

As malaria control efforts progress, the contribution of less common parasites like Plasmodium ovale to overall transmission becomes more significant.

Identifying and treating cases of Plasmodium ovale are crucial steps toward malaria elimination.

8. Research and Surveillance:

Ongoing research is essential to better understand Plasmodium ovale's biology, drug susceptibility, and transmission dynamics.

Surveillance efforts must be enhanced to detect and monitor the presence of Plasmodium ovale and other less common malaria parasites.

In the context of malaria eradication, Plasmodium ovale presents unique challenges due to its often-overlooked status. While P. falciparum and P. vivax have received more attention, addressing the role of Plasmodium ovale is vital for achieving malaria elimination goals. Comprehensive surveillance, accurate diagnosis, effective treatment, and ongoing research are all essential components of a holistic approach to combat this lesser-known malaria parasite and ultimately work toward a malaria-free world.

CHAPTER 12: CONCLUSION AND FUTURE DIRECTIONS

RECAPITULATING KEY INSIGHTS

As we wrap up our exploration of malaria research, strategies, and the quest for eradication, it's crucial to recapitulate the key insights we've gained along the way. Malaria is a complex, global challenge, and understanding its nuances is pivotal in our collective efforts to combat and ultimately eliminate this devastating disease. Here are the key takeaways:

1. Malaria's Impact on Humanity:

Malaria has plagued humanity for centuries, causing immense suffering, economic burden, and loss of life.

Vulnerable populations, particularly in sub-Saharan Africa, bear the brunt of the disease.

2. Multifaceted Nature of Malaria:

Malaria is caused by Plasmodium parasites, with P. falciparum and P. vivax being the most prevalent and virulent species.

Plasmodium ovale and other less common parasites also play significant roles in malaria dynamics.

3. Malaria Prevention and Control:

Strategies like insecticide-treated bed nets, indoor residual spraying, and antimalarial drugs have made significant strides in reducing malaria transmission and mortality.

The importance of community engagement, health system strengthening, and cross-border collaborations cannot be overstated.

4. Challenges in Diagnosis and Treatment:

Accurate and prompt diagnosis is critical for effective treatment.

Drug resistance, especially in P. falciparum, remains a significant challenge.

5. Malaria Elimination and Eradication:

Malaria elimination efforts focus on reducing transmission to a level where it is no longer a public health concern in specific regions.

Eradication, the ultimate goal, involves the complete global elimination of the disease.

6. Global Initiatives and Partnerships:

Collaborative efforts through initiatives like the Roll Back Malaria (RBM) Partnership, the Global Fund, and regional alliances are essential in driving progress.

7. Innovation and Research:

Ongoing research is vital for developing new tools, diagnostics, drugs, and vaccines.

Understanding mosquito behavior, parasite genetics, and host immune responses informs control strategies.

8. Community Stories and Personal Experiences:

Narratives from healthcare workers, researchers, and individuals affected by malaria underscore the human dimension of the disease and inspire hope and resilience.

9. Global Resilience and Dedication:

The global community's unwavering commitment to malaria control and eradication is evident through advocacy, funding, and cross-sectoral collaborations.

10. The Road Ahead:

- Malaria eradication is an ambitious but attainable goal that requires persistence, innovation, and collaboration.

- The fight against malaria remains a priority on the global health agenda, with the aim of creating a world free from the burden of this preventable and treatable disease.

It is clear that the battle against malaria is far from over. However, the progress made, the lessons learned, and the dedication of individuals, organizations, and governments offer hope for a future where malaria is no longer a threat to our world. This journey reminds us of the power of collective action and the resilience of the human spirit in the face of one of humanity's oldest foes.

THE CONTINUING QUEST TO UNDERSTAND PLASMODIUM OVALE

Plasmodium ovale, often overshadowed by its more infamous malaria parasite counterparts, continues to intrigue researchers and scientists as they seek to unravel its mysteries. Understanding the biology, epidemiology, and clinical implications of Plasmodium ovale is crucial for comprehensive malaria control and elimination efforts. Here, we delve into the ongoing quest to understand this lesser-known malaria parasite:

1. Unmasking Plasmodium Ovale's Diversity:

Recent genetic studies have revealed that Plasmodium ovale consists of two distinct species, P. ovale curtisi and P. ovale wallikeri. Recognizing this diversity is essential for tailored control measures.

2. Geographic Distribution and Prevalence:

Plasmodium ovale is found in regions across sub-Saharan Africa, Southeast Asia, and the Western Pacific.

Its prevalence varies within and between countries, making it a challenging target for malaria control.

3. Clinical Profiles and Symptomatology:

Plasmodium ovale infections typically present with fever, chills, and other malaria-like symptoms.

Understanding the clinical spectrum, severity, and complications of P. ovale is essential for timely diagnosis and treatment.

4. Relapsing Malaria:

Plasmodium ovale shares a unique trait with P. vivax—it can cause relapsing malaria. Dormant liver-stage parasites can lead to recurrent infections months or even years after the initial infection.

5. Diagnosis Challenges:

Plasmodium ovale's resemblance to P. vivax in blood smears can lead to misdiagnosis, impacting treatment.

Molecular and genetic diagnostics are increasingly used to differentiate between these species.

6. Antimalarial Drug Susceptibility:

Plasmodium ovale has demonstrated resistance to certain antimalarial drugs, necessitating alternative treatment approaches.

Monitoring its drug susceptibility patterns is essential for effective case management.

7. Potential Roles in Transmission:

Research is ongoing to determine Plasmodium ovale's contribution to malaria transmission.

Understanding its role in sustaining the parasite reservoir is critical for elimination efforts.

8. Host Immune Responses:

Investigating how the human immune system responds to Plasmodium ovale infections can inform vaccine development and treatment strategies.

9. Vector Behavior and Transmission:

Understanding the behavior and preferences of mosquito vectors that transmit Plasmodium ovale is essential for targeted vector control measures.

10. Integrated Research Approaches:

- Cross-disciplinary collaboration, including genetic, clinical, epidemiological, and entomological research, is vital for a comprehensive understanding of Plasmodium ovale.

11. Impact on Malaria Control Goals:

- Plasmodium ovale's prevalence and unique characteristics may influence malaria control and elimination strategies.

- Its contribution to the overall malaria burden underscores the importance of recognizing and addressing this lesser-known parasite.

As the quest to understand Plasmodium ovale continues, researchers and scientists remain dedicated to unlocking its secrets. Comprehensive knowledge of this parasite's biology, epidemiology, and clinical manifestations is essential for tailoring effective malaria control measures, improving diagnostics, and advancing drug and vaccine development.

In this journey, the enigmatic Plasmodium ovale serves as a reminder of the complexity of malaria and the ongoing commitment to eliminating this global health threat.

A CALL TO ACTION: UNITING AGAINST MALARIA

Malaria, a preventable and treatable disease, continues to pose a significant global health challenge, affecting millions of people annually. Despite the progress made in reducing malaria-related deaths and transmission, much work remains to be done. The fight against malaria requires a concerted effort from individuals, communities, governments, organizations, and the international community. Here is a call to action to unite against malaria:

1. Increase Awareness and Education:

Raise awareness about malaria's impact on individuals, families, and communities.

Educate people about the importance of malaria prevention, early diagnosis, and prompt treatment.

2. Advocate for Funding:

Advocate for increased funding for malaria control and elimination efforts at the national and international levels.

Ensure that resources are allocated efficiently to reach vulnerable populations.

3. Strengthen Health Systems:

Invest in robust healthcare systems to improve access to malaria diagnosis and treatment in underserved areas.

Train and support healthcare workers to deliver quality care and treatment.

4. Innovate for Solutions:

Support research and innovation to develop new tools, including diagnostics, drugs, and vaccines, to combat malaria.

Explore novel vector control strategies and technologies to reduce mosquito-borne transmission.

5. Community Engagement:

Empower communities to take ownership of malaria control efforts by engaging them in prevention activities and education.

Mobilize community health workers to reach remote and at-risk populations.

6. Cross-Border Collaboration:

Foster collaboration between neighboring countries to address cross-border transmission and harmonize control efforts.

Share best practices, research findings, and resources to strengthen regional malaria control.

7. Malaria-Free Schools and Workplaces:

Promote malaria prevention in schools and workplaces, ensuring that children and employees are protected from the disease.

Encourage corporate social responsibility initiatives to support malaria control.

8. Advocate for Policy Change:

Advocate for policies that prioritize malaria control and elimination as part of broader public health agendas.

Ensure that policies align with international guidelines and best practices.

9. Support Vulnerable Populations:

- Target interventions to protect vulnerable populations, such as pregnant women, children under five, and displaced communities.

- Ensure that marginalized groups have access to healthcare services.

10. Measure Progress and Accountability:

- Establish clear metrics and monitoring mechanisms to track progress toward malaria control and elimination goals.

- Hold governments and organizations accountable for their commitments and responsibilities.

11. Mobilize Global Solidarity:

- Recognize that malaria is a global issue that requires international cooperation.

- Partner with organizations, governments, and stakeholders worldwide to pool resources and expertise.

12. Work Toward Eradication:

- Embrace the long-term vision of malaria eradication and invest in strategies that move us closer to this goal.

- Recognize that eradicating malaria will bring substantial economic and health benefits.

13. Personal Responsibility:

- Individuals can take steps to protect themselves from malaria, such as using bed nets, seeking early diagnosis, and adhering to treatment.

- Travelers to malaria-endemic areas should take preventive measures and follow recommended guidelines.

Malaria is a preventable and treatable disease, and with collective action, we can make significant strides toward its control and eventual eradication. It is a call to action for governments, organizations, communities, and individuals to unite against malaria, working together to save lives, reduce suffering, and build a healthier, malaria-free world.

CONCLUSION

In the pages of "Exploring Plasmodium Ovale – A Comprehensive Guide to Malaria's Lesser-Known Culprit," we embarked on a journey of discovery, unearthing the complexities of a malaria parasite often overlooked but undeniably significant. Authored by Tom Wiles, this comprehensive guide has been a beacon of knowledge, shedding light on Plasmodium ovale and its role in the grand narrative of malaria.

We began by peering into the historical annals of malaria research, tracing the footsteps of dedicated scientists and researchers who unraveled the mysteries of this ancient disease. From its historical origins to the modern-day quest for eradication, we grasped the enormity of the challenge and the relentless determination of those who have pursued solutions.

The book then led us through the intricate life cycle of Plasmodium ovale, exposing its unique attributes and the challenges it presents in diagnosis, treatment, and control. We delved into the significance of this lesser-known culprit in malaria epidemiology and its implications for global health.

We embarked on a voyage across continents, exploring the global distribution patterns of Plasmodium ovale and the factors influencing its geographic prevalence. We contemplated the symbiotic relationship between mosquito hosts and human hosts, recognizing the intricate dance that perpetuates malaria transmission.

As we delved deeper into differentiating Plasmodium ovale from other malaria parasites, we unveiled the importance of accurate diagnosis and the consequences of misclassification. Genomic discoveries and genetic variability provided insights into the parasite's evolution and adaptation.

The shadow of drug resistance loomed, and we confronted the implications of this formidable challenge in our battle against malaria. We acknowledged the indispensable role of molecular biology in unraveling the secrets of Plasmodium ovale.

Transmission pathways and vector biology illuminated the path forward in vector control efforts, while surveillance strategies and epidemiological studies became our guiding lights in the darkness of uncertainty.

With a clear vision, we explored targeted interventions for Plasmodium ovale control and contemplated the past, present, and future of antimalarial therapies. We dissected the challenges in treating Plasmodium ovale infections and embraced case management strategies and guidelines as beacons of hope.

In our quest, we observed the intricate dance between the parasite and the human immune system, uncovering immune evasion mechanisms and the potential for vaccine development. We celebrated ongoing research initiatives and innovations as the torchbearers of progress.

Advances in diagnostic tools and techniques offered a glimpse of a brighter future, while promising avenues for future discoveries beckoned us forward. We heard the narratives of malaria researchers and healthcare workers, their voices resounding with dedication and resilience.

We listened to personal experiences in battling malaria, where stories of survival and triumph over adversity reaffirmed our commitment to the cause.

As we conclude this comprehensive guide, authored by Tom Wiles, we are left with a profound sense of the work that lies ahead. Malaria, with Plasmodium ovale as one of its enigmatic players, remains a formidable adversary. Yet, armed with knowledge, innovation, and unwavering dedication, we stand united against this ancient scourge.

This book is not merely a collection of words on pages; it is a call to action. It beckons us to join hands, across borders and boundaries, to continue the unceasing quest to conquer malaria. Together, we have the power to illuminate the darkness, uncover the secrets of Plasmodium ovale, and forge a path toward a world where malaria is but a distant memory—a world where health, hope, and resilience prevail.

www.ingramcontent.com/pod-product-compliance
Lightning Source LLC
Chambersburg PA
CBHW070930260726
48661CB00003B/911